21

The A–Z Reference Book of Childhood Conditions

Patricia Gilbert

Clinical Tutor and Senior Lecturer
University of Warwick
UK

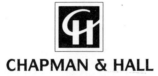

CHAPMAN & HALL

London · Glasgow · Weinheim · New York · Tokyo · Melbourne · Madras

Published by Chapman & Hall, 2–6 Boundary Row, London SE1 8HN, UK

Chapman & Hall, 2–6 Boundary Row, London SE1 8HN, UK

Blackie Academic & Professional, Wester Cleddens Road, Bishopbriggs, Glasgow G64 2NZ, UK

Chapman & Hall GmbH, Pappelallee 3, 69469 Weinheim, Germany

Chapman & Hall USA, One Penn Plaza, 41st Floor, New York NY 10119, USA

Chapman & Hall Japan, ITP-Japan, Kyowa Building, 3F, 2-2-1 Hirakawacho, Chiyoda-ku, Tokyo 102, Japan

Chapman & Hall Australia, Thomas Nelson Australia, 102 Dodds Street, South Melbourne, Victoria 3205, Australia

Chapman & Hall India, R. Seshadri, 32 Second Main Road, CIT East, Madras 600 035, India

First edition 1995

© 1995 Patricia Gilbert

This edition not for sale in North America and Australia; orders from these regions should be referred to Singular Publishing Group, Inc., 4284 41st Street, San Diego, CA92105, USA

Typeset in 10/12 Times by Mews Photosetting, Beckenham, Kent
Printed in England by Clays Ltd, St Ives plc, Suffolk

ISBN 0 412 57470 5

A catalogue record for this book is available from the British Library

∞ Printed on permanent acid-free text paper, manufactured in accordance with the proposed ANSI/NISO Z39.48-1992 and ANSI/NISO Z39.48-1984 (Permanence of Paper).

Contents

Preface

Children, as well as adults, become ill. Any time or place can herald the onset of sometimes severe or even life-threatening illness. For instance, a child may set off for school seemingly perfectly fit and well. But by midday the child can be burning with fever, in severe pain or maybe in need of urgent hospital admission.

Anyone having the care of children, and certainly those many dedicated people who spend their lives working with children, need a basic knowledge of childhood illnesses. As well as knowledge of emergency treatment for a variety of conditions, knowledge of prevention and the spread of infectious disease, as well as the natural history of the illness, is valuable in the working situation. Teachers, play-group leaders, nursery staff, social workers as well as those people more intimately concerned with the care of sick children need a quick, ready reference for unexpected events that may occur during the course of a working day. Parents, including the many devoted foster-parents having the care of a number of children throughout their lives, can also require a readily available source of reference.

It is hoped that this volume will prove of value in this context. The alphabetical arrangement facilitates rapid access to the appropriate condition. The index is also comprehensively arranged to allow for specific symptoms to lead the reader to the most likely cause of the problem.

Long-term implications as well as possible later complications are also to be found under the appropriate heading. The emphasis is on the practical day-to-day management of the many common – and some less common – illnesses affecting children.

Selection of the conditions included has been based on two criteria. Firstly, the condition under discussion is relatively common, and one from which many children will suffer during the course of their early lives. This includes the common infectious illnesses such as gastroenteritis, chickenpox and tonsillitis, for example, as well as such diverse conditions as bed-wetting, warts and eczema. Secondly, the condition is less common, but is one which it is important to understand in order that the child can be helped to lead as normal a life as is possible within the limitations of the condition. This group includes such conditions as diabetes, epilepsy and coeliac disease as well as other possibly less well-known conditions such as Perthes' disease and epidermolysis bullosa. All these conditions can be found amongst both schoolchildren and their younger brothers and sisters.

A glossary of some unavoidable medical terms has been added at the end of the book and, where appropriate, names and addresses of self-help groups have been added at the end of each specific section. Statistics on the incidence levels of infectious diseases have been taken from data in HMSO publications.

It is hoped that this book will be a valuable 'working companion' to the many people who have the vital day-to-day care of the up-and-coming generation.

Acknowledgements

My thanks are due, once again, to Dr Terry Billington for the superb work done in reading this manuscript. Her comments and suggestions have been gratefully received, but any errors are entirely my own.

Rosemary Morris at Chapman & Hall has been generous with encouragement over the past months, and her ever-willing availability for discussion has been of enormous assistance in the completion of this volume.

As ever, my wider thanks are due to the many children and their parents who, over the years, have allowed me into their homes and lives when problems of health have arisen.

Special features of children's diseases

Children are not 'mini-adults'. They are special people in their own right with special problems and needs. This is probably never so obvious as when they become ill.

PATTERNS OF ILLNESS

These, in everyone, can be broken down into five basic causative factors.

Disease (or 'lack of ease') can be due to a **congenital** problem. This includes all the multitude of syndromes, more and more of which are being recognized, described and classified with every passing week. A congenital disease is one which is present from birth, and which has its roots in a genetic or chromosomal defect. These defects may be inherited from either parent or can be the result of a mutation during cell division. Examples of these types of problems can range from the serious to the relatively minor. For example, Down's syndrome is the result of a chromosomal rearrangement, the results of which have far-ranging effects for the child and family throughout life. A further example of a congenital disorder is haemophilia, in which direct family links can be followed. This disease affects only males, but is passed on through the female line. As with Down's syndrome, the effects of this congenital problem are felt throughout life.

Relatively minor congenital problems can also occur such as, for example, webbing of the toes, or an extra digit on one hand. (Look in old paintings for the long sleeves that hide the sixth digit on Anne Boleyn's hand!) These latter findings are unlikely to cause any significant problems in later life, but make a fascinating part of the study of family history.

Many of the congenital problems are obvious either at birth or certainly during the first few weeks of life. With accurate diagnosis and sensitive long-term advice and discussion, parents can be helped to come to terms with their child's congenital condition. Also, of great importance, they can be shown ways to help their child grow to reach his or her full potential with the help of other people concerned with the care of the child, nursery staff and teachers bringing their own special expertise.

Secondly, **infections** of all kinds play a large part in the illness of children. Newborn babies arrive in the world with some immunity to the infectious agents which surround us all the time. This immunity is passed on from mother to child both prenatally and in breast-milk, provided, of course, that the mother herself has contracted and overcome the specific disease. For example, if a mother has never suffered an attack of measles (but remember that attacks of infection can be subclinical) she will have no antibodies available in her body to pass on to her baby. So the baby will be susceptible to this infection should it be met. As the baby grows and matures, immunity to infectious disease will be gained. But to do this the child will, of necessity, have to suffer from the infection. This gaining of natural immunity makes up a large part of the illnesses of childhood.

Before the advent of **active immunization**, against a number of infections, many children were laid low – and sometimes with fatal results – by these so-called 'childhood infections'. Today's children in the western world are fortunate indeed to have the vaccines available to prevent the large-scale epidemics (which occurred with monotonous regularity) of such diseases as diphtheria and polio and, until fairly recently, measles, mumps and rubella. But infections such as sore throats, headaches and runny noses still abound, and lucky are the children – and their parents – who escape with only a few of these episodes in the pre-school and early school years. Unfortunately, unlike the childhood infections such as mumps and chickenpox, the bacteria/viruses causing the common cold undergo subtle changes every year or so. Hence the immunity gained one year against one specific type of infection is not effective against the infections occurring the following year. Thus the seemingly endless round of upper respiratory tract infections persists throughout the early years of childhood.

Other more serious forms of infection, such as meningitis, are also hazards to be remembered when a child becomes ill. Immunization has recently become available against one particular form of meningitis. But there are a number of other infective agents that can cause this serious disease.

Again, today's children are fortunate that powerful antibiotics are available to be used in the fight against infectious disease. But these drugs are effective only against bacterial infections (with very few exceptions). Infections with viruses are not helped by antibiotics.

So, infections of all kinds probably account for much of the illness during the childhood years. And, in spite of modern medicine and treatments, long-term complications – and fatalities – do still occur.

New growths or **tumours** can also cause illness in children as well as in adult life. Cancers of all kinds affect children, leukaemia (a cancer of the blood) perhaps being the commonest and most well-known of these. The types of tumours encountered in childhood differ from the adult pattern. Some are similar, but there are a number of cancers which are specific to childhood, such as Wilm's tumour and retinoblastoma.

This group of illnesses must always be remembered when a child is ill for an unusually long time. They are now second only to accidents as a cause of death in the 1–15-year age group. Quick diagnosis and treatment in these circumstances must be undertaken for the best chance of cure.

The fourth main category of disease comprises the **degenerative** diseases. These are far more commonly seen in the older generation, but occasionally children are affected by these types of conditions. Examples of these are the degenerative brain disorders such as the mucopolysaccharide diseases – Hunter's and Hurler's syndromes – and other conditions with a biochemical basis. Many of these diseases have a genetic basis, and must always be remembered if a child, of school age or during the toddler years, shows a fall-off of skills that have already been learned.

Finally, **allergic disease** is a common cause of illness in childhood. Examples of these types of disorders are asthma, eczema and hay-fever – so often seen in one form or another in members of the same family. In this group can also be placed certain types of food allergy, such as the allergy to the protein in wheat seen in children (and adults) with coeliac disease. Allergy to cow's milk (often a temporary phase only) as well as other food allergies are also important aspects of childhood illness.

(**Accidents** of all kinds, from accidental poisoning to road traffic accidents, are a further important cause of distress and 'dis-ease' in children. Their cause, prevention and treatment form a subject on their own.)

TYPES OF DISEASE

As has already been hinted at, these can be quite different from those in adults and specific to the childhood years. The osteochondrites in which certain bones (Perthes' disease affecting the hips, for example) become weakened and friable, causing pain and loss of use, are good examples of this. No such condition is seen in adult life. The specific tumours – Wilm's tumour and retinoblastoma – are further examples of conditions found only in childhood.

Further pitfalls in diagnosis can also arise in the ways in which children **react** to disease. For instance, an adult with tonsillitis will be only too well aware of a sore throat being the basic reason for feeling unwell. A child with a similar condition can easily throw a mother off the scent by complaining of abdominal pain, and make no mention at all of a sore throat even though this can be a fiery red and very obviously infected. Maybe this is because the child has not developed, as yet, the verbal skills to accurately pinpoint the pain, or maybe it is because different physiological patterns occur in childhood. Whatever the reason, the knowledge of these factors will enable the true diagnosis to be made (and hence appropriate treatment given) more rapidly.

Children also react to disease, such as an infection, more rapidly than do adults. All child-carers are aware that children can wake perfectly fit and bubbling over with life and energy, but by lunch-time they can be feverish, in pain and, on occasions, severely ill. Fortunately the reverse also holds true. Children can bounce back to health in a surprisingly short time.

STAGE OF DEVELOPMENT

The stage of development reached when a child suffers a specific disease is also of importance when the long-term effects are being considered. For example, a severe infection of one kind or another contracted during the early stage of speech development can cause marked delay in the acquisition of this skill. If a similar infection is acquired at a much later date – 10 years of age or so when speech and language are fully developed – there will be little or no effect on this skill.

Similarly a child's other developmental 'milestones' such as the motor one of walking and the finer motor skills, such as hand dexterity, can be affected more seriously by an illness during the critical months of development of the particular skill.

All in all, disease in children can be a minefield of diagnostic pitfalls! But how satisfying and rewarding can be the results of correct detection of the clues, leading to appropriate treatment and cure of many of the childhood ills. Heart-ache too, can regretfully occur when a disease is found to be, in the present state of knowledge, incurable. But at least the child's life can be made as comfortable and fulfilling as possible by accurate knowledge of the natural history and course of the condition.

Acne

INCIDENCE

The exact incidence of acne is not documented. But the condition is so common in adolescence as to be almost a normal part of growing-up. Fortunate indeed are the adolescents who escape with no signs of acne at all. Boys are more commonly affected than girls.

Whilst adolescence is by far the most usual time of life for acne to occur, newborn babies are occasionally seen with the typical lesions, usually on the cheeks. No treatment is necessary at this early age, as the acne will disappear spontaneously by around 6 weeks.

Again, acne can make its first appearance at around 3 months of age, also most often only on the cheeks. At this age it can be more of a persistent problem, and will need treatment if it is to clear within the next 2 years. Often there is a strong family history of acne, and these children frequently have a return of the typical rash later in life, most commonly in the adolescent years.

HISTORY

Acne has been described in the literature from time immemorial. The word 'acne' comes from the Greek word 'acme', meaning the pinnacle, or prime, of life. An apt description of adolesence – physically at least!

CAUSATION

The rash of acne arises from the sebaceous glands. The commonest areas of the body to be affected are the face, back and chest. The sebaceous glands secrete a substance known as sebum. This substance largely consists of fatty chemicals which perform the vital function of lubricating the skin. With the appearance of acne, a number of changes take place in these glands, as follows.

- There is an increase in the amount of sebum produced.
- There is an increase in the fatty acid content of the sebum.

- The lining of the ducts become thickened to produce the typical comedones (or 'blackheads') of acne. (The blackening is due to an increase in pigment, and not due to dirt!)
- A specific type of bacterium causes inflammation to occur around the glands.

These changes, occurring in varying degrees in different people, give rise to the typical rash of acne.

There are a number of underlying factors which, in turn, cause these changes to take place, as follows.

- At puberty there is an increase in the male **hormones**, especially in boys. Girls also have a proportion of male hormone in their bodies, and at puberty there can be a temporary imbalance in the proportions of male and female hormones.
- In girls, **fluid retention** can be a problem premenstrually. This is thought to have a bearing on the worsening of acne during the premenstrual days.

These two factors are the most important causes of acne, the temporary hormonal imbalance being the most important. Other factors include the following.

- Certain items of **diet** have been said to affect the severity of the lesions in some boys and girls. Chocolate, coffee and nuts have all been implicated, but this is an individual variation.
- Some specific **oils** used in certain industries – and even the oil used in some cosmetics – can lead to a worsening of the rash. DDT and some weedkillers have also been implicated in the onset of acne.
- **Drugs**, such as the steroids, some anticonvulsant drugs and some of the combined types of oral contraceptives, can also be triggering causes.
- The **time of year** also appers to have a bearing on the severity of the rash, summer light having a good effect. Acne is often at its worst during the winter months.

CHARACTERISTICS

There are two main types of acne described, in addition to the type seen in young children.

Acne vulgaris is by far the most common type. Around 40% of boys have some degree of this type of acne between 17 and 19 years of age. Girls seem to suffer from acne at a slightly earlier age – around 16 to 18 years – probably coinciding with the optimum time of hormonal imbalance.

The skin of sufferers often tends to be more greasy than normal, due to the increased production of sebum. In severe cases the rash can leave scars which remain visible throughout life, the scars seen on the back of the neck in some adult men being a permanent reminder of their youth.

Acne conglobata is a severe form of acne in which the spots are so numerous that they become confluent, with many inflamed and cystic nodules filled with pus. In extreme cases there can be associated fever and general feelings of ill-health. This is especially common in the tropics.

MANAGEMENT

This can require long-term sensitive handling during the adolescent years when it is important – for both boys and girls – to look as good as possible. They should be reassured that their spots will eventually clear, but meanwhile there are a number of treatments that can be tried.

It is important to keep the skin as **clean** as possible to reduce the incidence of infection of the spots with the bacteria specific to acne. Holding a hot damp flannel to the face – or bending over a bowl of steaming water – will open up the pores. If this is followed by gentle washing with unperfumed soap, infection will be reduced to a minimum. This should be done two or three times a day.

There are a number of **proprietary preparations** on the market for application to the rash for the control of acne. Most of these act by dissolving the plug of dried skin cells in the spots (or comedones) as well as reducing the greasiness of the skin.

Vitamin A, manufactured as a cream, can also be helpful.

Sunlight has a beneficial effect on acne. Ultraviolet light has been tried as a treatment, but is found to be less effective than natural sunlight. But it is useful in the winter months when natural sunlight is at a minimum.

Oxytetracycline, or **erythromycin**, in tablet form, is also helpful in some severe cases of acne. It is often necessary to take this form of medication on a long-term basis (several months) before any improvement is seen. (The tetracycline interferes with the action of some forms of contraceptive pill and must not be given in pregnancy. So care must be taken with this form of treatment in adolescent girls.)

Other medicants are available to treat extremely severe cases of acne. These must be given with care, and very carefully monitored, as serious side-effects can occur.

A number of ways of controlling the condition may have to be tried before finding a treatment that suits the individual person with acne. Reassurance that the rash will eventually disappear is an all-important ingredient in the treatment. It must be stressed that any treatment given must be continued on a long-term basis.

PREVENTION

There is no known prevention for acne, apart from choosing to be born into a family that has no history of acne! Scrupulous cleanliness of the affected areas, and persistence with treatment, are the best ways of controlling the condition.

THE FUTURE

Acne in adulthood is rare, although it is thought that around 1% of men and 5% of women have some degree of acne in middle life.

Anorexia nervosa

Alternative name

Eating disorder.

INCIDENCE

Anorexia nervosa is most commonly found in adolescent girls. But the condition is by no means unknown in younger children. Also, in a recent survey it was found that one-quarter of the cases in this younger age group were boys.

In the younger age group (8–14 years of age) the condition can reach a dangerous state without recognition, probably due to the fact that anorexia nervosa is considered to be solely a disease of older girls.

The incidence of this condition appears to be on the increase in western countries.

CAUSATION

This is difficult to define precisely, as there can be many factors involved. In adolescent girls psychological factors are probably the prime instigators in the onset of anorexia nervosa. Today's fashions all shout the message that 'thin is beautiful', and the fashion-conscious teenager will respond to this. Anorexia sufferers also have a distorted image of their own body shape, insisting that they are fat, ugly and 'overweight', when, in fact, their bones stand out starkly and unattractively.

At a deeper level, it is possible that fear of adulthood with all its responsibilities and stresses can subconsciously lead the adolescent into ways of keeping a childish anatomy and physiology. The menarche – around 12–14 years – is a definitive sign of approaching maturity, and this is the age when anorexia commonly begins.

Overly close family relationships are also considered to have a possible bearing on the aetiology of anorexia nervosa. This especially applies to a close, intrusive mother–daughter relationship. Children with this condition also tend to be perfectionists who worry about many aspects of everyday living.

CHARACTERISTICS

The onset of anorexia nervosa is usually insidious, youngsters using all kinds of tactics so that parents will be unaware of how little they are eating. Food is hidden, small helpings are frequently requested, meals are avoided, strange diets are tried and, later in the disease, the sufferer will induce vomiting and/or use excessive doses of laxatives.

The physical features of this disease are very non-specific. It is when these features are combined with other behavioural abnormalities that anorexia nervosa should be suspected.

Physical characteristics

Weight loss: this, of course, is the most important sign. In children during the actively growing years, it must be remembered that **lack** of normal **weight gain** is also a significant factor. The ratios of the weight and height for age must be taken into consideration.

Obvious **lack of appetite**: most children from 8 years upwards have healthy appetites, unless they are suffering from a concurrent infection or some other disorder. A transient anorexia often follows such events, but usually soon picks up again.

After a long day at school, or pursuing some other holiday activity, the evening meal is generally consumed with relish. Children with anorexia will make all kinds of excuses for avoiding this meal, as follows:

- The child may complain of **abdominal pain or discomfort**, and may make this an excuse for not eating.
- Complaints of **tiredness** and **dizziness** may also be features of this condition.

On examination of the child, features other than thinness and a poor weight (in relation to age and height) are seen:

- **cold hands and feet** due to poor circulation;
- a **dry skin**;
- a **low blood pressure**;
- a **slow pulse**, and, later on in the disease, **slow, deep breathing**.

(In late stages of the disease the child's breath will have the characteristic smell of acetone (pear-drops). This is due to the breakdown of body tissue as a result of the virtual starvation.)

Behavioural characteristics

- There is **moodiness** with depressive thoughts and outlook.
- There is **loss of interest** in most aspects of living, including activities previously much enjoyed.
- There is often a marked interest in some aspects of **food**, including such emotive issues as animal rights and hunger in the world.
- There may be a **clinical depression** in association with these other manifestations of anorexia nervosa. On the opposite side of the coin, some children can cope extraordinarily well for some time. This is especially true of 'highfliers', who often manage to keep up high examination standards.

Bulimia nervosa is an allied condition, and can coexist with anorexia nervosa. Here the sufferer will 'binge', or overeat, and then induce vomiting. Excessive purgatives can also be taken in an effort to counteract the overeating.

Ultimately, when fluids are being refused as well as food, **dehydration** can occur. Signs of this serious condition are sunken eyes, a weak pulse, a low blood pressure and a decreased output of urine. The child is then seriously ill and in urgent need of treatment.

Death can occur – and does in around 5% of children with severe anorexia nervosa. Death can be due either to hypothermia, an infection which the weakened body is unable to counteract or to irreversible changes in the body chemistry.

MANAGEMENT

Treatment for severe anorexia nervosa is difficult and long-term. Often a period of hospital admission – preferably in a specialized unit – is needed. The initial aim is to **rehydrate** and **refeed** the child until a normal pattern of eating has been re-established. This obviously cannot happen overnight – the child who has eaten practically nothing will need to increase intake at a slow, but steady, rate. The help of a dietician is valuable in ensuring a balanced diet. In very severe cases, where the child is determined not to eat, nasogastric feeding may need to be undertaken as a last resort during the initial stages of treatment. (Occasionally, the suggestion that this might be done is sufficient to start the child eating again.)

Once this initial physical hurdle has been overcome, it is necessary for the basic cause of the original onset of the anorexia to be tackled. A child psychiatrist with a special interest in anorexic children is of prime importance in the liaison which must take place between paediatrician, general practitioner, health visitor, dietician and others concerned with helping the child and the family.

Treatment for any underlying depressive disease with antidepressant drugs must also be undertaken.

THE FUTURE

A **return** of the anorexia nervosa at times of stress – examinations, boy–girl relationships etc. – can occur, and must be contained by early specialized help.

Depending at what stage of growth the anorexia has occurred, **final adult height** may be adversely affected. This is particularly likely to happen if the condition has occurred during the time of a growth spurt.

Later, **fertility** may be affected in girls. This is due to the possibilty of changes to the ovaries and uterus during the time of poor nutrition. The incidence of this effect is not fully known.

Osteoporosis is also thought to be a possible late effect of earlier anorexia nervosa. The early teenage years are a time when a healthy bony skeleton is laid down. If virtual starvation at this time precludes this, adequate later bone density may be poor. Again, this effect is not fully understood.

Anorexia nervosa can be a difficult condition to, first of all, diagnose, and, secondly, to treat. Best results are obtained with early help before body changes become too pronounced or severe.

SELF-HELP GROUP

The Eating Disorder Association
Sackville Place
44–48 Magdalen Street
Norwich
Norfolk NR3 1JE
(Tel. 0603 621414)

Appendicitis

INCIDENCE

Appendicitis is no more common in childhood than in adult life. A recent national survey in Britain found that around 3 or 4 children in every 1000 suffered from appendicitis every year. The condition is seen at any age, but is more usually found over the age of 5 years. Appendicitis is an emergency at any age, but especially so in children. The appendix is a small, finger-like projection from the caecum – a part of the large intestine situated in the right lower part of the abdomen. In childhood the wall of this vestigial organ is thin, and so rupture can occur more readily. Rupture leads to **peritonitis**. This is a serious condition where the abdominal cavity becomes inflamed and infected due to the contents of the bowel spilling out into this body cavity. Unless the appendix is removed surgically the condition can be fatal. In fact, there were four deaths from appendicitis in Scotland as recently as the late 1970s.

HISTORY

Probably the most well-known historical fact related to appendicitis is King Edward VII's appendicectomy. This operation, way back in the early days of the twentieth century, was one of the first to be successfully performed in Britain.

CAUSATION

In plant-eating animals, the appendix fulfils a digestive function. In the human this organ is merely a vestigial remnant, fulfilling no useful purpose at all. Inflammation occurs in this part of the intestine with specific bacteria which are normally present. It is when either a kink develops in the appendix itself or something obstructs the lumen that problems can arise. The offending obstruction can be anything from, for example, an apple-pip to a toothbrush bristle! More frequently, however, hardened food material is found to be the probable cause of the obstruction.

Initially the inflammation is localized in the appendix, but surrounding lymph glands and other abdominal tissues quickly become involved. It is this reaction that gives rise to the typical pain of appendicitis.

CHARACTERISTICS

The correct diagnosis of acute abdominal pain in children is notoriously difficult. Appendicitis can be just one of the many causes of this common childhood symptom. Much experience is necessary to unravel all the clues. But it is vital that an acute inflammation of the appendix is not missed. In fact, it is preferable for a normal appendix to be removed than for an inflamed – and potentially dangerous – one to be missed.

Typically, the signs of appendicitis are as follows.

- There is a sudden onset (over an hour or so) of **colicky abdominal pain**. This pain can be continuous, or alternatively come in spasms. The pain usually starts around the area of the umbilicus. In adults, the pain typically moves, after a short time, to the right lower part of the abdomen. This can also occur in children, but frequently the child describes the main pain as remaining in the centre of the abdomen. If the appendix is in an unusual position behind the main bowel, the pain is felt more in the loin region.
- Most children with appendicitis have at least one episode of **vomiting**.
- **Diarrhoea** is also a relatively common feature at first in childhood appendicitis. This is then followed by constipation.
- There is commonly, but not invariably, a rise in **temperature**.
- The child will prefer to **lie still** and curled round in an attempt to reduce the pain.

INVESTIGATIONS

There are no specific investigations that need to be made to confirm the diagnosis of appendicitis, although **ultrasound scans** may be used as an aid to diagnosis. It is, however, wise to **test the child's urine** to exclude a urinary infection as the cause of the pain.

MANAGEMENT

The treatment for appendicitis is an operation to remove the appendix. Even if, at operation, the appendix is found not to be inflamed, it is removed to prevent trouble at any later date. A short stay in hospital is necessary following surgery. If the child has been seriously ill prior to operation, intravenous fluids may be necessary for a short while during, and after, the operation. Dissolvable stitches are used, so that there need be no fear for the child of their removal – as was the case a decade or so ago.

Early **movement** is encouraged, and the child should be allowed to play. Children are very good at judging the limits of their abilities under such circumstances.

A normal **diet** can be given as soon as the child asks for food.

Schooling can usually be resumed after 2 or 3 weeks following an appendicectomy. This will depend, of course, on how ill the child has been prior to surgery. No restrictions need to be put on activities, but any complaints of pain after physical activities should always be fully investigated, and quieter pursuits advised for a short time.

COMPLICATIONS

There are few complications to a straightforward appendicectomy, but occasionally **infection** can occur locally around the incision. This is readily cured with antibiotics.

THE FUTURE

There are no long-term problems following appendicitis. Indeed, if the appendix has been removed, appendicitis need never again be considered as a possible cause of future abdominal pain!

Arthritis

Alternative names

Juvenile chronic arthritis (the name most commonly used).
Juvenile rheumatoid arthritis.
Still's disease.
(Both the two latter names are rarely used. This follows review of
the classification of this disease, necessary because of the wide
variations in manifestations of the disease.)

INCIDENCE

There are no exact figures available for the incidence of juvenile chronic arthritis, but it is probably the most common of the connective disorders seen in childhood. It is seen in all countries of the world, and is thought probably to have an incidence similar to that of diabetes in childhood, i.e. around 2 children in every 1000 suffering from the disease. So whilst it is not a particularly common disease, affected children will need much monitoring and care.

The usual age of onset is below 5 years, but the condition can occur in any age group throughout childhood. Both sexes are equally affected.

(This form of rheumatic arthritis must not be confused with acute rheumatic fever, which was a far more common, and serious, disease of childhood half a century or so ago. Acute rheumatic fever is also primarily a disease of connective tissue, and can have arthritis as part of its symptomatology. There is a strong association between acute rheumatic fever and infection with a particular type of streptococcal bacterium which is not the case with juvenile chronic arthritis. The incidence of rheumatic fever has declined due to three factors:

1. better living conditions which diminish infection rates;
2. the advent of the penicillins which are active against the streptococcal bacterium;
3. a decline in the virulence of the specific streptococcal bacterium.)

HISTORY

It was Dr George Frederic Still who first described the condition (or group of conditions) now known as juvenile chronic arthritis in 1896. Until fairly recently the condition was referred to as 'Still's disease'. It is since the specific subtypes have been classified more stringently that the disease has been referred to as juvenile chronic arthritis.

CAUSATION

Juvenile chronic arthritis is part of the wide group of diseases which affect the connective tissues of the body. Several factors are thought to be involved in the causation of the disease – firstly, there is probably some genetic predisposition to this group of diseases; secondly, there is an auto-immune process (in which the body starts attacking its own tissues); and, finally, added infection may play a part in the onset.

CHARACTERISTICS

Arthritis and rheumatism are wide-ranging disorders of connective tissue, there being over 200 different types known. Several of these can affect children. Three of the more common modes of onset, and subsequent progress, of the disease will be described.

Systemic juvenile chronic arthritis

This type of arthritis begins with a feverish illness. The **fever** occurs daily and can be as high as 40.5°C. This fever usually resolves at some time during the day, only to return again within the next 24 hours. This intermittent pattern can make the diagnosis difficult to differentiate from a number of other diseases which have an intermittent fever as part of the initial symptomatology.

All the attendant signs and symptoms associated with fever occur – a **rapid pulse**, **shivery feelings**, **lack of appetite** and **irritability**.

Glands in the neck, armpit and groin become swollen and tender.

A **rash**, of a typical coppery-red colour, also affects some children during these initial stages of the illness. This rash is especially noticeable following a hot bath, but is not an irritating one. At this early stage, **arthritis** with tender swollen joints may be completely absent – only to appear a few weeks, or even months, later. (This fact can, of course, make for great difficulties in diagnosis.)

Investigations for systemic onset disease

Whilst there are no specific tests for juvenile chronic arthritis, **blood tests** will show abnormalities, as follows.

- The **white blood cell count** is high.
- **Anaemia** is usually present.
- The **erythrocyte sedimentation rate** (ESR) is raised. (This is a non-specific test which is positive in any condition where there is any degree of inflammation, due to any cause.

All these findings can be due to any number of other conditions, and so are of no specific help in diagnosis, but, of course, all give added clues.

To add to the difficulties, a positive rheumatoid factor, found in the blood in other types of onset of this disease, is rarely found when the disease has this acute systemic onset.

Polyarticular juvenile chronic arthritis

This is perhaps an easier onset from the diagnostic point of view, for the following reasons.

- A number of **joints** will be **painful**, **red** and **swollen**. The joints involved in this process are usually the smaller ones of the body – wrists, finger joints, ankles and, at times, knees. The specialized joints in the neck (those with limited movement) can also be involved. Due to this the child may complain of neck pain, and may be holding the head over to one side. The temporomandibular joint (concerned with opening the jaw) is also often involved. For this type of juvenile chronic arthritis to be diagnosed, five or more joints should be involved in the disease process.
- A **low grade fever** can also be present, but is quite unlike the variable, spiking fever pattern associated with the acute systemic onset of the condition.
- Swelling of the **lymph glands** may also occur, but not to such a marked extent as with the systemic type onset.

Investigations for polyarticular disease

A **blood test** specific for the rheumatoid factor can be done, but again can be somewhat unhelpful – some children will have a positive rheumatoid factor, but by no means all! It is important, however, that this test is done, as those children who have a positive reading do not have such a good future outlook as those children who do not have this positive finding in their blood.

Pauciarticular juvenile chronic arthritis

This type of arthritis is diagnosed when four, or fewer, joints are involved in the disease process. Over half of the children with juvenile chronic arthritis fall into this group. Symptoms include the following.

- There is **pain, redness,** and **swelling** of one – or up to four – joints of the body. It is the knees and ankles that are most frequently affected in this subgroup of arthritis.
- Children with this type of juvenile arthritis have **none of the generalized effects** seen in the other two subgroups. They remain generally well, with no fever, throughout the course of the illness.

MANAGEMENT

Adequate **rest** is an important factor in the treatment of children with juvenile chronic arthritis. Complete bed rest is only necessary for those children seriously ill with the disease – namely, those children with the serious system type or with many painfully affected joints. But all children with the condition will benefit from an adequate night's rest – around 12 hours every night is a good working figure, and if not actually sleeping, at least resting in bed. An hour or two's rest in the middle of the day is also advisable.

Physiotherapy plays an important part in the treatment of juvenile arthritis. Once the most acutely painful stage of joint involvement is over, an exercise programme tailored to the individual needs of the child should be planned. The aim is twofold:

1. to maintain the mobility of the joints;
2. to keep up the strength of the muscles around the joints.

Hydrotherapy pools are valuable for these treatments. The warm water makes painful joints easier to move, and also the buoyancy afforded by the water makes exercising muscles less stressful. The aim is to put all joints of the body through a full range of movement every day.

Splinting of joints is also an important part of treatment. During the acutely painful stages of the disease, specially fitted splints should be worn at night to prevent deformity occurring. These will have the added benefit of relief of pain when joints can be inadvertently moved during sleep. During the day, splints can give relief from pain when worn over joints in constant use – such as, for example, wrists during a school day.

The **drug** treatment of juvenile arthritis is complex and is dependent upon the type and severity of the disease in each individual child.

Aspirin, or one of the many other non-steroidal drugs, is the first type of drug to be used. Each individual child will need careful monitoring, both for the benefit from the drug and for the unwanted side-effects that occur when many drugs are prescribed.

Second-line drugs include **gold** and **penicillamine** preparations. Again, these must be carefully prescribed and monitored by doctors specializing in the treatment of juvenile arthritis.

Finally **steroid** drugs are used if treatment with the other types of drug is not controlling the disease. The decision to use long-term steroids is one that must not be taken lightly, due to the serious side-effects that can result from prolonged use of these drugs. In children, retardation of growth, as a side-effect, is an ever-present worry.

Mixtures of all these drugs, tailored to each child's specific needs, can be used.

Local steroid injections into specific joints can give short-term relief and prevent total loss of function in the joint in selected cases.

Schooling can be continued once the acute stage of the disease (as in the systemic onset type) is over. Limitations on physical activities will need to be sorted out between educational and health staff. Generally speaking, competitive sports such as football, hockey and sprinting are not suitable. Even if the child feels able to compete, energies should be tactfully diverted into other activities more suitable for potentially damaged joints. For example, swimming as a sport is one in which the child with juvenile arthritis should be able to keep up with peers. Also, as a leisure activity, cycling is suitable. (It is advisable to be sure that the atlantoaxial joint – at the base of the skull – is stable before commencing any sport.)

For children with severe disease, **special schooling** may be necessary.

Occupational therapists can also provide valuable help for the severely affected child who has difficulty with such everyday activities as dressing, toileting or eating. Much help can also be given to provide suitable activities when long periods of bed rest become necessary for children severely affected by the disease.

COMPLICATIONS

Complications affecting the **eye** are the only ones in parts of the body other than the joints. Here, a condition known as iridocyclitis can occur. Long-term inflammation of different parts of the eye can lead to cataract formation and/or glaucoma. These latter effects are seen more frequently in children having the pauciarticular type of juvenile chronic arthritis. Surgical treatment for cataracts may be necessary at a later date, and glaucoma may need surgical or drug treatment.

Complications can also occur due to the necessity for **long-term drug treatment**, especially if the steroid drugs have to be used for any length of time. **Slowing of growth** can occur under these circumstances together with an increased susceptibility to **infections** of all kinds. **Osteoporosis** (thinning of the bones) can also be a result of the long-term use of steroids, as well as resulting from the disease itself.

THE FUTURE

Juvenile chronic arthritis is a long-term disease, and the future will depend on both the type of disease and the response to treatment. Some children will be severely handicapped throughout life by their arthritis. They may need later surgery to replace disorganized and useless, painful joints or to release tight muscles which are causing deformity. But 70–80% of sufferers will lead useful, independent lives.

For less severe manifestations of the arthritis, adequate splinting during exacerbations of the disease will do much to keep deformity to a minimum. Physiotherapy, on a long-term basis, is also vital to preserve mobility of joints and muscle strength.

SELF-HELP GROUPS

Children's Chronic Arthritis Association
47 Battenhall Avenue
Worcester WR5 2HN
(Tel. 0905 763556)

Lady Hoare Trust for Physically Disabled Children
44–46 Fleet Street
London EC4Y 1BN
(Tel. 071 583 1951)

Young Arthritis Care
18 Stephenson Way
London NW1 2HD
(Tel. 071 916 1500)

Asthma

INCIDENCE

It is difficult to quote the exact incidence of asthma, partly due to the problems with the precise definition of this condition. The interface between 'wheezy' bronchitis and asthma has been blurred, making for difficulties in quantifying the disease.

Recently, figures for school children in Britain with asthma have been quoted as being as high as 1 in 4. A research project has shown that 1 in every 7 children takes an inhaler to school to use if they feel an attack of asthma is imminent. So, if the condition is underdiagnosed and treatment other than with inhalers is taken into account, the figure of 25% may not be so far from the truth.

There are other reports pointing to an increasing incidence of asthma, such as:

- eight thousand emergency severe asthma admissions every year to hospitals in one region of Britain;
- a figure of 1.7 million children in Britain suffering from some degree of asthma;
- two thousand deaths occuring every year in Britain as a result of asthma, 50 children under the age of 15 years included in this figure.

So it would appear that, as well as being a relatively common condition, asthma is increasing in incidence in Britain. But on the 'up' side, it is thought that half of the children suffering from asthma will stop having attacks when they are adults.

The severity of the asthma varies greatly. This ranges from the child who has infrequent attacks with no need to stay away from school, to the child who needs an inhaler nearby at all times. This latter child may also need frequent hospital admissions to deal with severe life-threatening attacks.

Boys are affected twice as frequently as girls by this condition.

There is also often a strong family history of allergies of one kind or another. It is thought that around half of the children suffering from severe asthma have someone else in the family who has either asthma, eczema, hay-fever or some other form of specific allergy.

Asthma seems to be less troublesome during the winter months. It has been found that the highest incidence of hospital admissions with asthma was between May and June and between September and November. These times of the year, of course, correspond to the optimum times of allergic substances in nature.

Asthma is known world-wide – only in the rural areas of developing countries is the disease rare. The highest rates of increase are seen in the advanced civilizations of the world. It is this fact that leads to the conclusion that environmental factors have a strong influence on the incidence of asthma.

HISTORY

William Osler, the well-known Canadian physician who was a professor of medicine in Oxford during the last century, considered asthma to be a 'neurotic disorder'. Half a century on, this view had undergone a marked change, with asthma being recognized as a distinct clinical entity, with treatment for attacks being routinely prescribed.

In the late 1960s Dr Roger Altounyan, a physician deeply interested in immunology, discovered the action of the drugs which today are used to prevent asthma attacks.

CAUSATION

Both heredity and environment are causative factors in asthma.

Hereditary factors, as mentioned previously, play a part in determining whether a child suffers from asthma. Any child whose parents or siblings have one of the atopic allergic problems is more likely to be asthmatic than a child who has no such family history. ('Atopy' can be described as any allergic condition in which specific antibodies are produced in response to a variety of outside stimuli. These include such conditions as hay-fever, eczema, allergic rhinitis and allergic conjunctivitis.)

The **environmental factors** that can be involved in the onset of an attack of asthma are legion. They are usually specific to each sufferer, although frequently more than one substance, or a group of substances, can initiate an attack.

Probably one of the commonest allergens (those substances to which a child reacts) is the common **house dust mite**. These are the minute creatures which inhabit the houses – and especially the beds – of even the cleanest and most hygienic of dwellings. This probably accounts for the large number of night-time attacks of asthma. (It is now known that the season of late summer/early autumn in Britain is the time when the house-dust mites are at their most numerous. This possibly accounts for the increase in asthma during the months of September to November.)

Dogs, cats, horses and other furry creatures affect many children. This effectively precludes them from beneficial contact with domestic pets and other animals.

Feathers in pillows can cause attacks of wheezing in susceptible children.

A smoky atmosphere in a house where adults **smoke** is also a potent factor in the onset of an asthmatic attack.

External factors such as **pollen** from trees and flowers in springtime can be the triggering factor for many children. Media reports of pollen counts in various parts of the country can alert asthma sufferers to take extra precautionary measures.

In recent years, **air pollutants** in cities from exhaust fumes of cars and lorries have been postulated as a possible cause for the increase in asthma. It is thought that this form of air pollution does not in itself cause asthma, but enhances the allergic response in susceptible people, including children. Microscopic particles from diesel oil have also been implicated, but this has yet to be clarified.

Infections of the upper respiratory tract by viruses are also implicated in the onset of an attack of asthma (infections due to bacteria are not thought to produce such a response). This causative factor is thought to be of special importance in children who seem very prone to infections of this kind.

Intolerance to certain **foods** has been considered to be a factor. This is difficult to prove either way, conclusively, although some parents are quite certain that some foods – specific to each individual child – will bring on an attack of asthma.

Exercise, particularly in cold air, will tend to exacerbate asthma in some children. If it is warm and humid outside, an attack of asthma is not so likely to occur. The warm humid atmospheres of swimming baths rarely bring on an attack for this reason.

Psychological factors in some children can be a causative trigger. Excitement, or worry, can result in an attack. Even laughter can precipitate a short-lived wheezy attack, as can crying.

There are thus many possible triggering factors to be looked at when treatment for an asthmatic child is being considered!

CHARACTERISTICS

In children, asthma as a diagnosis should be considered if the following are found.

- **Wheezy breathing** is heard under specific, but isolated, conditions. Examples of the onset of this symptom are: during the course of a viral respiratory infection; on exercise, especially outside on a cold winter's day; when the pollen count is high. There are plenty of other examples, each dependent on the individual susceptibility of each child.

- The child has a **cough** and especially so if this occurs frequently during the night.
- This night-time cough is associated with **breathlessness**.
- On **physical examination** there is often little to be learned from listening to the child's chest, particularly if this is done between the attacks of wheeziness. The main use of this form of examination is to exclude other reasons for the wheezy attacks, which will give specific findings.
- A **diary** kept by the child's mother showing when asthmatic attacks occur in relationship to exercise or exposure to any of the other well-known trigger factors is of great value, both in helping to make the diagnosis and in planning treatment.
- In severe, long-standing cases of asthma there can be **poor growth** and **chest deformity**.

It may seem strange that these relatively few features occur with such a common, and potentially serious, condition. This is partly why the diagnosis of asthma can be so difficult. It is of interest to note what exactly is happening in the bronchi of the child with asthma:

- a narrowing of the bronchi by the action of the specific allergen on the tiny muscles in the walls of these structures;
- swelling of the mucosal lining of the bronchi;
- sticky secretions partially blocking the narrowed lumen of the bronchi.

When all these three abnormalities occur together, it is no wonder that the child has difficulty in breathing, the 'breathing out' part of the cycle being the one especially affected during an asthmatic attack.

INVESTIGATIONS

A chest **X-ray** is taken initially. This will not show any changes specific to asthma, but will exclude any other reasons for the child's attacks of wheeziness – such as, for example, something stuck in one of the bronchi. (It is amazing how long a peanut can remain stuck in a small child's bronchi, with only wheezy breathing to announce its presence.)

Taking readings from a **peak flow meter** is the most helpful investigation. These readings can vary at different times of the day, and also in relationship to physical activities.

Skin tests for allergic substances are of limited value. Any child with any allergic symptoms will probably react to most of the common allergens such as house mite dust, pollen or animal fur.

MANAGEMENT

This is a specialized subject, and in some parts of the country there are clinics devoted entirely to the management of asthma. Treatment will vary depending on both the frequency and severity of the attacks of asthma.

All parents of children with asthma should endeavour to identify, and remove as far as possible, the **triggering factors** in the household. For example, the household's **pet** may have to be found another home if contact with the susceptible child brings on asthma. Measures to reduce the amount of **house dust** are important. 'Damp dusting' can help, as can vacuuming of mattresses in an attempt to get rid of the house-dust mite. Synthetic fillings for pillows and cushions should be tried in case the child is allergic to feathers. (As an emergency measure for getting rid of the mite, try popping the pillows and duvets into the freezer for a while. The house-dust mite detests the cold!)

Smoking should be strongly discouraged if any family member has asthma. This rule should also apply to visitors to the house.

Sporting activities should not be discouraged. It is better to give children suitable medication so that they can take part in the school activities than to stop them taking part. (It can be a difficult balance to keep between over-protection of asthmatic children and allowing them to run the risk of severe asthmatic attacks. Parents should receive full **explanations** of their child's disease, along with advice on how to handle everyday activities and events.)

Schooling for asthmatic children should be along as normal lines as possible. Teachers should be aware of the child's respiratory problems and should know what action to take if an asthmatic attack should occur during the school day. Many children will need to take their inhalers – containing the medication that has been prescribed for them individually – to school. Easy, and quick, access to these inhalers is important for children who are too young to manage their medication for themselves.

Psychological factors such as anxiety and over-excitement should be reduced to a minimum. (Parents should be aware, however, of youngsters learning how to get their own way by working themselves up to initiate an attack of asthma.)

If there is thought to be any possible **food intolerance**, the potentially offending foods should be avoided.

Drug treatment

There are three main groups of drugs used in the treatment of asthma, as follows.

1. The **bronchodilator drugs**. This group of drugs acts by relaxing the muscles around the bronchi. It is the constriction of these muscles that causes the bronchi to narrow in response to an allergen in an attack of

asthma. The most commonly used drugs in this group are the ones that act on specific muscle receptors and are known as **beta-agonists**. They can either be taken by mouth, used as an inhaler or used in a nebulizer. The way in which these drugs are taken will depend on the age of the child and the severity of the asthma. These drugs are only available on prescription. (There are other different types of bronchodilator drugs available, but these can have problems with side-effects and so are rarely prescribed. Strangely enough, some of these drugs are available for sale by pharmacists without a prescription. It is very unwise to buy and give these drugs to children. **Always** contact your doctor if your child has a wheezy cough.).

2. The **corticosteroid drugs**. These drugs act mainly by their potent anti-inflammatory action. This means that the swelling and mucous secretions in the bronchi as a result of the allergic reaction are both reduced. These drugs can be taken either by mouth or by an inhaler. Side-effects can occur with corticosteroid drugs when taken by mouth if they are used on a long-term basis. One of the most important of these side-effects to control is the suppression of growth. Serious side-effects do not occur when these drugs are taken by inhaler, although infection with 'thrush' (a fungal infection) can occur in the child's mouth if the inhaler is used over any length of time.

3. The **non-steroidal drugs** which are used to prevent attacks of asthma. (These were the important drugs discovered by Dr Altounyan in the 1960s.) Sodium cromoglycate is the most frequently used drug in this group, and has revolutionized the treatment of asthma. It is used as an inhaler on a regular basis – usually four times a day – to prevent asthma. It can also be used immediately before undertaking any activity known to precipitate an attack – for example, horse-riding.

The drug treatment of asthma is a complicated one, needing constant review over the years. This is especially necessary for asthmatic children as the severity and pattern of their asthma can vary throughout the years of growth. Special asthma clinics are the ideal way to monitor the various possible drug regimes.

The treatment of an acute, life-threatening attack of asthma is very specialized. First aid measures will include the rapid giving of any specifically prescribed medicine, adequate fresh air, putting the child in the most comfortable position (usually sitting forward and leaning on a table) and calling the emergency services on a 999 call. Open access to the ward has proved to be very advantageous for the child with asthma.

Parents should be warned not to overemphasize their child's asthma.

THE FUTURE

Asthma is a condition that can burn itself out in childhood so that very few, if any, attacks are suffered in adulthood. This will apply to around half the individuals who have asthma during their childhood years. It is impossible to predict which child will continue to suffer from asthma throughout life. A strong family history of allergic disease is not an encouraging feature from this point of view.

SELF-HELP GROUPS

National Asthma Campaign
Providence House
Providence Place
London N1 0NT
(Tel. 071 226 2260)

This group has a number of useful leaflets available on all aspects of coping with asthma.

The British Lung Foundation
Kingsmead House
250 King's Road
London SW3 5UE
(Tel. 071 376 5735)

can also give helpful information.

Bronchitis

INCIDENCE

Bronchitis is a common condition, especially during the cold winter months. Much confusion has arisen – and still arises – over the differentiation of 'wheezy bronchitis' and asthma. (This is discussed further in the text under 'asthma'.) Bronchitis is an inflammation of the bronchi – the cartilaginous tubes leading from the trachea (windpipe) to the alveoli of the lung tissue. It is in these minute alveoli that the actual gaseous exchanges take place, and when infection reaches this part of the lung it is known as pneumonia.

Whilst children up to the age of 5 years suffer, on average, from around six upper respiratory tract infections every year, relatively few of them go on to suffer from bronchitis.

Teething and bronchitis together are a well-known facet of folklore. In reality there is no connection between this infection and the entirely normal process of cutting teeth. It is just possible that the pain and upset that some children suffer when their teeth are erupting can lower their resistance to infection. It is perhaps due to this aspect that bronchitis can sometimes occur at the same time as the teething process.

The incidence of bronchitis in older children is variable; a mild attack of bronchitis sometimes occurs with an upper respiratory infection. Those children who have recurrent 'wheezy' bronchitis are probably suffering from asthma.

CAUSATION

Bronchitis usually arises from a viral infection. These infections usually begin in the nose and throat, and then descend, in some children more frequently than others, to the lower respiratory tract. It is less usual for there to be a bacterial cause for bronchitis, although there can be added bacterial infection following on from an initial viral infection.

Measles and whooping cough – a viral and bacterial infection respectively – are always complicated by bronchitis to some degree.

CHARACTERISTICS

Bronchitis usually follows on from, or is seen in conjunction with, an upper respiratory tract infection, the symptoms of which are well known to everyone – a runny nose, sore throat and maybe a mild fever.

The one diagnostic symptom of bronchitis is a **cough**. This cough is dry in the early stages, but within a day or two will become loose, and yellowish **sputum** may be coughed up. Children, however, tend not to cough up secretions, but to swallow them. This can on occasions cause **vomiting**.

A **wheeze** can also be heard in some children with bronchitis. This is due to the narrowing of the bronchi as a result of the infection. (The wheeze is caused by the air passing through the narrowed passages.) But this, as mentioned previously, can also be a manifestation of asthma. There may be, but not invariably, a mild **fever** together with general feelings of **malaise**. The child may also be reluctant to eat.

On listening to the child's chest with a stethoscope, the typical sounds of the air passing through the inflamed bronchi can be heard.

MANAGEMENT

In a straightforward case of bronchitis, antibiotics are of no value, as the infection is usually viral in origin. (Antibiotics have no action against viruses.) A light **diet**, with plenty of **fluids** (of the child's preference), with play in a warm room is all the treatment that is necessary.

If the cough becomes excessively irritant, keeping the child – and the rest of the family – awake at night, a soothing **linctus** can be given. A mixture containing glycerine, honey and lemon is suitable, and can be obtained from pharmacists. (Other proprietary cough mixtures, many of which have a cough suppressant action, are not advisable. The cough is part of the body's natural defence mechanism, being useful in removing infected material from the lower respiratory tract.)

If the child with bronchitis is particularly wheezy, medication to dilate the bronchi can be prescribed to good effect.

Attendance at **school** should cease until the worst of the cough has cleared, and the child is feeling able to cope with the physical demands of school again.

In an uncomplicated attack of bronchitis the cough will clear within a week to 10 days, and the child will return to full health.

COMPLICATIONS

Secondary bacterial infection of the bronchi can occur. Under these circumstances, the cough will be showing no signs of improvement, and

and may even be worsening. The child may also become more feverish, or run a fever where there has been none before. Antibiotics will be needed to clear the infection under these conditions.

Pneumonia, where the infection reaches the alveoli of the lung, can be a complication of bronchitis. Again this infection can be due to either a virus or a bacterium. (Pneumonia can occur, of course, without a preceding upper respiratory tract infection or bronchitis. This is especially the case in premature babies, children who have some congenital defect or those children who are malnourished.)

The infection can affect either the whole of a lung (or both lungs) or a segment or lobe of a lung. The former is known as bronchopneumonia and the latter as segmental, or lobar, pneumonia.

The child with pneumonia will be seriously ill. There will be a rapid rate of respiration – this is in direct contrast to the picture seen with bronchitis where the respiratory rate is within normal limits. The nostrils will be dilated as the child struggles to get air into the lungs. The cough will be persistent and irritating, and fever will be high. This is altogether a far more severe set of symptoms than is seen with an attack of bronchitis.

Investigations if pneumonia is suspected include a chest X-ray and a throat swab and blood test to be examined in the laboratory for the infecting organism.

Hospital admission is necessary for the child severely ill with pneumonia. Nursing in an oxygen tent and intravenous fluids may be necessary during the initial acute stages. Antibiotics are necessary to cure the infection. Even if the initial pneumonia was caused by a virus, secondary infection with bacteria is common.

Older children with a less severe attack of pneumonia can be nursed at home if the home circumstances are suitable. Parents should always be encouraged to contact their doctor again if they are at all worried about their child's condition.

THE FUTURE

Uncomplicated bronchitis will have no permanent after-effects on the child. It is when the symptoms become blurred with those of asthma that long-term effects – due to the asthma – may occur.

Chickenpox

Alternative name

Varicella.

INCIDENCE

The exact incidence of attacks of chickenpox in children is not known. It is, however, a common and highly infectious disease occurring most usually in the 2–8-year age group. Chickenpox is found all over the world except in a few isolated communities. In children the disease is usually a mild one with few complications or permanent after-effects. In adults contracting the disease this picture can be different, serious illness occasionally being the result. So, from this point of view, it is preferable that chickenpox should be contracted during childhood. (Introduction of the infection to isolated communities who do not generally suffer from chickenpox can also be serious.) There are two groups of children in whom an attack of chickenpox can also have serious results. These are:

1. those who are receiving immunosuppressant drugs for some other condition;
2. very young babies.

In both these groups chickenpox can be a life-threatening disease. Hospital admission will be necessary for both these conditions.

CAUSATION

Chickenpox is caused by a virus. Immunity, gained by a naturally acquired attack of the disease, is usually life-long, so that second attacks are extremely rare. But it is not unusual for an attack of shingles to occur in later life, often following a period of general debility. This is due to a reawakening of the virus, which has lain dormant in the body for many years. On the other side of the coin, a child can contract chickenpox from a grandparent with shingles.

Chickenpox has an incubation period of 14–21 days with, most usually, the next member of the family showing signs of the infection on around the sixteenth day. The infection is most likely to be transmitted during the first few days of symptoms. The virus is then present in the saliva, so that droplet infection from the breath or during sneezing or coughing is the common mode of passage of the virus.

CHARACTERISTICS

The infection starts, in many children, with a mild non-specific illness with a general feeling of **malaise** and frequently a **low-grade fever**, **headache** and occasionally a **sore throat** – in fact very similar to the symptoms and signs of a common cold. It is not until the appearance of the typical **rash** that chickenpox can be said to be the cause of the original symptoms. The rash passes through three stages. Firstly, there is a raised, red, discrete rash which, within a very short time, will become blistery. It is at this stage that the diagnosis of chickenpox will become obvious. After 2 or 3 days, the clear fluid within the vesicle (or 'blister-like' spot) will become cloudy and of a yellowish colour. As the disease progresses, these spots will crust over, leaving a scab which, if scratched off, can leave a permanent white scar.

The rash appears in crops with 2 or 3 days between the appearance of each crop. Due to this 'cropping', the various stages of the rash can be seen at any one time.

The distribution of the rash of chickenpox is also very specific. Initially the rash is confined to the chest and face regions of the body, with covered areas of the body having more spots than exposed parts. By the third day, the rash spreads to the limbs. In mild cases relatively few spots occur. But in severe cases, the rash can be very extensive and even include the palms of the hands and the soles of the feet. In all but the very mildest of attacks, the rash is also found on the mucous membranes of the mouth and ears, and, in the most severe cases, in the eyes and the vagina.

Severe **irritation** is one of the most unpleasant aspects of chickenpox. This symptom makes its appearance soon after the vesicles have started to crust over. Scratching at this time can cause **scarring** to occur or, more seriously, **infection** of the spots with bacteria.

INVESTIGATIONS

As a general rule with an uncomplicated attack of chickenpox no specific investigations are necessary. The diagnosis is made on clinical grounds alone.

The virus can be isolated in the laboratory from the fluid in the vesicles during the first 3 or 4 days of the rash. But this is usually an unnecessary exercise, except in unusual cases where there is some doubt about the diagnosis.

MANAGEMENT

General sympathetic **care** is all that is needed for a mild, uncomplicated attack of chickenpox. A light **diet** with plenty of cool drinks is sensible during the early stages when the child is feeling generally unwell with a fever. Confinement to bed is unnecessary – quiet play in a warm room is all that is needed.

Calamine lotion and frequent **tepid baths** will do much to allay the irritation of chickenpox. If the itching is a problem in spite of this treatment, an **antihistamine cream** can be tried. Fingernails should be cut as short as possible to prevent injury through scratching.

Schooling can be resumed after 1 week from the onset of the rash **if** (and only if) the child is feeling perfectly well. Once the spots have crusted over, transmission of infection is no longer a problem – the scabs contain no active virus. Many children are sent home from school because they still have a few crusted spots. This is an unnecessary precaution from the transmission of infection point of view. It is only if children are still feeling unwell that they should be at home.

COMPLICATIONS

These are rare with an attack of chickenpox.

Secondary infection of the rash, due to scratching, is the most usual complication of this, mainly mild, disease of childhood. Antibiotics may be necessary if this is severe.

Pneumonia can occur in adults or immunosuppressed children with an attack of chickenpox. Children without other underlying disease will not suffer from this complication.

Encephalitis is a further possible, but rare, complication.

PREVENTION

There is at present no **immunization** available against chickenpox, although research into this possibility is taking place. With such a generally mild disease of childhood with few serious complications a vaccine for general use would seem to be unnecessary. For immunosuppressed and otherwise ill children, however, the picture is different and a vaccine to prevent the infection would be of use.

Quarantine measures are unlikely to succeed as chickenpox is such a highly infectious disorder at a time before the diagnosis becomes obvious.

THE FUTURE

There are generally no future problems following an attack of chickenpox. The only possibility is an attack of shingles later in life due to a reawakening of the dormant virus.

Coeliac disease

INCIDENCE

Coeliac disease appears to be predominantly a condition seen amongst people of European and American origin. Whilst it is not unknown in the Far East and Africa, the incidence does not appear to be as high as in America and Europe. This may, however, be due to differences in the recording of disease types. In Britain, the incidence is reported as being between 1 in 2000 and 1 in 6000 – quite a wide variation. (In Northern Ireland, the incidence has been said to be as high as 1 in 300.)

HISTORY

This condition was recognized in children over 100 years ago. But it was not until the early 1950s that the relationship between coeliac disease and the eating of wheat-flour products was noticed by a Dr Dicke. Later in the 1950s the pathological changes in the small intestine were described.

CAUSATION

Coeliac disease is one of the many malabsorption conditions found in both adults and children. There are a great number of these conditions – some mild, some serious, some temporary, some permanent – in which the malabsorption of food is the basic cause. Coeliac disease is one in which there is an allergic response of the small intestine to the substance gluten, which is found in wheat and wheat products. Some sufferers are also allergic to a similar substance found in barley, oats and their products. It is thought that there is a basic immunological fault in the individual with coeliac disease causing the pathological changes seen in the small intestine following the eating of gluten-containing products. There appears to be a high familial incidence, although no specific genetic link has, as yet, been found.

CHARACTERISTICS

The age at which an affected child will show signs of coeliac disease varies between 9 and 18 months. The onset follows fairly soon after the beginning of mixed feeding with the inevitable inclusion in the diet of wheat products.

There are two main ways in which coeliac disease manifests itself, as follows.

1. There can be a relatively acute onset with **diarrhoea, lack of appetite** and a marked **abdominal distension**. Over the succeeding weeks, there is a loss of weight. In the child with fully developed, untreated coeliac disease the contrast of the grossly distended tummy with the starkly thin buttocks and thighs is very marked.
2. There can be a slower, more insidious onset with signs of **lack of growth** both in **height** and **weight** and the development of an **iron-deficiency anaemia**. (The importance of serial measurements of height and weight, recorded on a centile chart, is highlighted once more in this condition.)

The child with coeliac disease will also tend to be miserable, and be complaining of tummy-ache and generally be off-colour.

INVESTIGATIONS

As well as the clinical and serial measurement signs noted, examination under the microscope of a small piece of the intestine is necessary to confirm the diagnosis. This is known as a **jejunal biopsy**, and relates to the specific part of the intestine, the jejunum, which is examined. This process is carried out by the child swallowing a special capsule – the Crosby capsule. This tiny instrument removes a small part of the intestine. The capsule is then recovered later from a bowel motion.

On examination under the microscope, the appearance of the lining of the small intestine is quite characteristic if coeliac disease is present. The normal picture is of a series of 'ridges' in the membrane. This makes for a large surface area through which absorption of food materials can occur. In coeliac disease these 'ridges' (in adults these structures are more finger-like and are known as 'villi') are completely absent. The result of this is that very little food can be absorbed.

Specific **blood tests** for iron and a specific antibody against gliadin (the protein in the gluten) can help with the diagnosis, as can measurement of the **fat excreted** in the motions. But these tests are non-specific, and can also be positive in other diseases of the small intestine. So it is always advisable to perform a jejunal biopsy before treatment is started. Ideally, a further jejunal biopsy should be done after several months on a gluten-free diet, when the microscopic picture of the small intestine will be seen to have returned to normal.

MANAGEMENT

The treatment for coeliac disease is a **gluten-free diet**. Within a few weeks a vast improvement will be seen in young sufferers. They will begin to gain weight, the diarrhoea (if this has been a problem) will cease, they will have more energy and they will be altogether happier, easier-to-manage children.

At first sight, the exclusion of all wheat-containing foods from the diet can seem daunting. But with advice from a dietician, and help and encouragement from the Coeliac Society, mothers and child-carers will soon become used to the new regime. In the light of present knowledge, a gluten-free diet should be adhered to for life.

It is vital that the child with coeliac disease should have **regular reviews** to be sure that normal growth and development are being maintained. At these reviews any problems with diet can also be ironed out.

Some authorities advise a **gluten challenge** after 2 or 3 years on the gluten-free diet. Wheat-containing foods are reintroduced into the diet and a further jejunal biopsy is performed. If the appearances under the microscope have regressed to the pre-gluten-free diet type, the diagnosis of coeliac disease is 100% correct. A further reason for performing these serial jejunal biopsies is to be sure that the gluten intolerance is permanent and not a transient phenomenon.

Children in whom the diagnosis has been delayed may need **dietary supplements** of vitamins and minerals for a short time until these important substances are able to be properly absorbed again. Specifically, the absorption of the mineral iron and vitamins D and K can be especially affected.

COMPLICATIONS

These are unusual, but if they do occur are readily rectified.

An **iron-deficiency anaemia** can occur in children in whom the diagnosis is delayed or difficult. Iron by mouth or injection will readily cure this.

Rickets due to lack of vitamin D absorption can also occur very occasionally if the diagnosis is delayed for any reason. Here again, vitamin D supplements will halt this process.

During the difficult period of **adolescence** strict adherence to the gluten-free diet may be less than perfect! No adolescent wishes to be eating different foods from their contemporaries and they often rebel against advice. Initially only minimal effects are seen, but eventually there will be a return of the malabsorption symptoms. Sensitive handling during this period can reduce problems to a minimum. (Perhaps this is hardly a 'complication', but nevertheless it is a situation which frequently occurs and one to be remembered during the adolescent years.)

THE FUTURE

There has been a reported increase in the incidence of intestinal cancer in people with coeliac disease, but this has not been fully elucidated. Also, it is not entirely clear whether strict adherence to a gluten-free diet throughout life has any bearing on this future possibility.

SELF-HELP GROUP

The Coeliac Society
PO Box 220
High Wycombe
Bucks HP11 2HY
(Tel. 0494 437278)

Constipation

Constipation is not a disease entity, but rather a symptom which can be associated with a wide range of conditions. But most frequently, chronic or long-term constipation is the result of an acute event (again due to any number of possible causes) which results in temporary constipation. This symptom is included in this book because of its relatively common occurrence and the concern it can cause both children and their parents. Early diagnosis of the cause followed by appropriate treatment is vital for the wellbeing of the whole family.

INCIDENCE

Constipation is not an exciting enough condition for anyone to want to measure the exact incidence. Nevertheless it is unusual for any outpatient paediatric clinic to go by without at least one child being seen for chronic constipation.

Constipation can be defined as delay in the passage of stools which can reach a chronic state in which the lower bowel is blocked by hard, bulky faeces.

CAUSATION

Causes of constipation are multiple. There are, however, certain groups of conditions which predispose to this symptom, as follows.

- There may be some abnormality in the intestine such as, for example, Hirschsprung's disease (in which there is a much narrowed segment of the intestine) or some gross narrowing around the anal region.
- Conditions in which children are forced into inactivity due to their physical condition can predispose to chronic constipation. Examples of this are cerebral palsy, spina bifida and hypothyroidism.
- An illness in which there has been a high fever can mean that the child has become dehydrated and/or eaten little food. Both these facts will contribute to constipation which, unless recognized and treated, can become a long-term problem.

- The presence of an anal fissure, in which there is a tiny crack in the skin around the anus, can make defaecation so painful as to put the child off going to the toilet completely! Stools will deliberately be held back. This has the effect of making the faeces hard and bulky and so even more painful to pass. In addition the lower bowel will become so stretched that eventually all normal sensation of the need to defaecate will be lost. So a vicious circle is set up.
- Unsympathetic rigid handling of toilet training in the toddler years can result in the child becoming desperately concerned about this normal bodily function. If this is also followed by inadequate toiletting facilities at nursery or school the problem is compounded.
- It is thought that intolerance to certain foods can be a causative factor in the onset of chronic constipation. This fact has always to be considered in a child who also has eczema or asthma.

There are thus many problems that could be causative factors in the onset of long-term constipation!

CHARACTERISTICS

(The characteristics described will be of long-term constipation and its treatment. The possible underlying causes – outlined above – will also need to be understood and treated.) The constipated child will often be brought to the surgery with the parents complaining that the child has **diarrhoea!** This can seem paradoxical, but can be understood when it is remembered that hard faeces are blocking the lower bowel tightly. The fluid waste-products above this blockage will gradually leak and be responsible for soiling the child's underwear, so making the parents think that diarrhoea is the cause of the problem.

On examining the child's abdomen the hardened faeces can easily be felt. On rectal examination, these solid masses can also easily be felt.

As the problem progresses so will the urge to have the bowels open diminish due to the over-stretching of the lower bowel. This, of course, compounds the problem. Occasionally the child will complain of abdominal pain when chronically constipated. But, surprisingly enough, this is not a common complaint.

INVESTIGATIONS

It is not often necessary to do any further investigations other than the initial examination. But occasionally an X-ray of the abdomen will show the extent of the constipation. (This can also be useful in verifying the diagnosis to the parents, who, after all, initially brought their child along with diarrhoea!)

MANAGEMENT

Treatment of any underlying cause for the constipation must be the long-term aim to prevent the condition recurring.

Dietary advice, preferably from a paediatric dietician, regarding adequate fluid and fibre intake, is vital.

Treatment of any **anal fissure** with a local anaesthetic cream is also of importance. A good result of emptying the bowel can often be achieved when pain is no longer felt on defaecation. Initially to empty the bowel completely, it is usually necessary to give two or more **enemas**. This can be done at the child's home, but it is often more satisfactory to admit the child to hospital for a day or two so that it can be certain that the bowel is completely clear. Following this a daily dose of a **laxative** should be given to be sure that the bowels are opened at least once a day. (A stool softener such as lactulose can be used in conjunction with a stimulant such as senna.) The dosage of the laxative drugs may need to be altered until the right amount is found to produce the desired result without giving the child diarrhoea. This medication will need to be continued until the bowel has been 're-educated'. With the gross overstretching by the hard mass of faeces for some considerable length of time the child will no longer be aware of the need to visit the lavatory. But as the rectum returns to its normal diameter, normal sensation will return.

Advice on **regular** – relaxed – **times** for visiting the toilet must be given, and practised, alongside the medical treatment. Immediately after breakfast is a good time (if an adequate period of time can be found at this often stressful time of the day). Food in the stomach can initiate the 'gastrocolic' reflex, which helps with bowel elimination.

A system of **star charts** can sometimes be helpful (as with enuresis – see elsewhere in the book). The child is encouraged to note on the chart the days when the bowels have been successfully opened. Emphasis must always be placed on success, rather than note taken of failure.

This regime will have to be continued for some considerable time before full success is achieved – months rather than weeks. Both parent and child can become disheartened by this need for lengthy treatment. So it is important that adequate **support** is given throughout this time by all involved – general practitioners, health visitors, clinic staff and dieticians.

In the event of no – or little – success over a considerable period of time, there may be need for **further investigation** to be sure that there is no anatomical, or other, abnormality that is giving rise to the chronic constipation.

Also, it is worth checking that the child has no hidden **fears** of visiting the toilet.

THE FUTURE

This is, of course, dependent upon the basic cause of the constipation in childhood. If there is no underlying abnormality, constipation need no longer be a problem in later life as long as a suitable diet and regular bowel movements are made a part of everyday living.

Deafness

Deafness of itself is not a disease entity. It can be a symptom of many types of disorder ranging from congenital and inherited problems to infections of all kinds and also injuries. There are two types of deafness – **sensorineural** deafness, in which the actual nerves of hearing are involved, and **conductive** deafness, in which there is interference in the passage of the sound waves to the nerves of hearing. These two types will be dealt with separately as, although the outcome – deafness – is the same, aetiology and treatment differ.

SENSORINEURAL DEAFNESS

INCIDENCE

A sensorineural hearing loss affects around 1 in every 1000 children. This figure includes those children who have a severe hearing loss – in the range 65–80 dB (decibels) – and those with a profound hearing loss – in the range of 85 dB and above.

CAUSATION

There are several possible causative factors for this type of deafness as follows.

- **Genetic:** deafness can be inherited in a number of ways – either as a dominant or a recessive characteristic, or, in some circumstances, in a sex-linked manner. Certain specific syndromes also have deafness as part of the symptomatology, for example Waardenburg's syndrome, Usher's syndrome and Treacher–Collins syndrome. (See *A–Z Reference Book of Syndromes and Inherited Disorders* by P. Gilbert, published by Chapman & Hall, for descriptions of these, and other, syndromes.)
- **Infective causes:** these can be infections acquired both prenatally and after birth. Infection during pregnancy can be with the cytomegalovirus, toxoplasmosis or (probably the most well-known of all) rubella. If any of

these infections are contracted at a critical time in pregnancy, during the development of the organs of hearing, a congenital deafness can result. Infections contracted during childhood can also have deafness occurring as a complication. Examples of such infections include measles, mumps and bacterial meningitis.

- Problems during the **neonatal period** (the first 4 weeks of life), such as jaundice or oxygen deficiency, can result in a sensorineural deafness.
- Certain **drugs** can also be a causative factor. Streptomycin used to be a fairly frequent cause of deafness, and a few antibiotics, given long term, must be watched for this side-effect. Drugs given during pregnancy can also be the culprits, thalidamide being the most well known. Quinine given during pregnancy is also known to have a possible similar effect.

CHARACTERISTICS

It is vital that a sensorineural deafness in babies is diagnosed as soon as possible. With a severe sensorineural hearing loss from birth the child will not be able to develop 'inner language' and so will never be able, in later life, to use language adequately. Checks for hearing are done routinely in Britain at 7–8 months of age. In some areas of the country, the 'acoustic cradle' is used to check the hearing of all newborn babies. A further check-list was introduced, in 1988, for parents themselves to check their baby's hearing at regular intervals throughout the early months of life.

It is important that any queries voiced by mothers regarding their baby's hearing should be carefully investigated and followed up. Mothers have an instinctive knowledge of problems before they are fully obvious to other people.

Babies at greater risk of deafness due to a strong **family history** of poor hearing must also be checked carefully.

Vision should also be watched throughout the child's early life in cases where the cause of the deafness is uncertain. Usher's syndrome, in which there are associated visual problems, can be the reason for the deafness, for example.

MANAGEMENT

Once the extent of the hearing loss has been determined, a plan of continuing treatment and education will need to be formulated. For children with a bilateral loss, **amplification** will be necessary to make full use of any residual hearing they may have. Radio transmission aids are the most successful.

Help from the services for the **hearing-impaired** can give much help and advice to minimize the child's handicap. This assistance will need to be continued for many years.

Many children can be happily integrated into ordinary **schools** with this form of help. A few especially handicapped children will need special schooling and/or teaching by 'signing'. (The most appropriate and successful method for teaching such children is hotly debated in educational circles. It would seem that an amalgam of all possible methods of communication would be the most satisfactory.)

Any associated handicap – such as, for example, the later visual problems seen in Usher's syndrome – must be assessed and managed appropriately.

With specialized – and early – teaching, children deaf from birth can develop understandable **speech**. The importance of early intervention cannot be stressed too highly.

THE FUTURE

Career choices must, of necessity, be severely curtailed for children with profound sensorineural hearing loss. Good careers advice should be available from the early teenage years onwards.

Later, when a **pregnancy** is contemplated, genetic counselling should be available for the prospective parents.

CONDUCTIVE DEAFNESS

INCIDENCE

This is by far the commonest cause of deafness in children. It is thought to affect around one-third of all children at one time or another between the ages of 2 and 5 years. Although many of these will improve within a few months, up to one-fifth of the affected children will have a hearing loss which persists into late childhood.

Both boys and girls are affected.

CAUSATION

The most usual cause of a conductive deafness is a secretory otitis media. This can occur following an acute attack of middle ear infection. In this condition, sticky fluid fills the cavity of the middle ear, which contains three tiny bones intimately concerned with the hearing process. (Secretory otitis media is frequently referred to as 'glue ear' due to the glue-like nature of the fluid in the middle ear.) Because of this fluid the ossicles in the middle ear are unable to work adequately. As a result of this, the movements of the tympanic membrane (the eardrum) are restricted, so dulling hearing.

The reason why this fluid persists in the middle ear following an attack of acute otitis media is thought to be due to lack of drainage of fluid away from the middle ear. Normally secretions are drained away from the middle ear into the back of the throat via a tiny tube – the Eustachian tube. Following an infection, this tube becomes blocked due either to swelling of the tissues or by mucus. Young children are especially prone to this, partly due to the relative frequency of upper respiratory tract infections and partly due to the small bore of the Eustachian tube in this age group.

CHARACTERISTICS

The child with a chronic secretory otitis media will often have a deafness of around 20–40 dB. This loss, however, may not be consistent, but fluctuate from week to week. This fact can easily mislead parents into thinking that their child is just 'not attending' during the periods when hearing is less than perfect. Even routine hearing tests may, at times, fail to pick up the hearing loss if the test is performed on a good day.

But even this relatively mild degree of hearing loss can interfere with the **acquisition of speech** in the younger age groups. Speech is learned by imitation of sounds heard, so if some specific frequencies are missed by the child – due to the hearing loss – fully comprehensive speech is attained with difficulty.

In the older child, who has just started school, for example, **behaviour problems** or periods of 'switching off' can occur. Problems such as these can result from the failure to hear instructions adequately – the child compensating, in other ways, for the failure in hearing. ('Switching off' for short periods can easily be confused with petit mal (see 'Epilepsy') unless the possibility of a hearing loss is remembered and checked on.) Children with a conductive deafness can also be thought to be **slow learners** if the hearing problem is not recognized and treated appropriately.

INVESTIGATIONS

Clinical examination of the ears of a child suspected of being deaf due to secretory otitis media can show a range of abnormalities on the eardrum. The drum can be seen to be pulled inwards and/or be of an unusual greyish colour. There may also be dilated blood vessels coursing across the eardrum. The advice of an ear, nose and throat surgeon will be needed in certain children with a view to further treatment.

Audiology tests, suitable for the age of the child, will give information as to the degree of the hearing loss. Under the age of 3 years distraction tests will be needed. After this age most children will be able to cope with pure-tone audiometric tests.

Impedance audiometry can also be used, in especially difficult cases, to determine hearing loss. (This test measures the minute movements of the ear-drum in response to sound by means of a special instrument held against the eardrum.)

MANAGEMENT

The best way to treat secretory otitis media which is causing a conductive deafness is controversial. The type of treatment an individual child will receive will depend on the views current in that part of the country. There are three main ways in which the child's hearing can be improved, as follows.

1. **Antihistamine drugs**, given by mouth, were previously thought to help reduce swelling around the Eustachian tube, and hence improve the drainage of the middle ear. Along with this treatment decongestant nasal drops were prescribed for the same purpose. Latter-day thinking is that this form of treatment is of little value.
2. An operative procedure – a **myringotomy** – can be performed. In this procedure, the eardrum is pierced (under a general anaesthetic) and the sticky fluid withdrawn. In addition to the removal of this fluid, tiny ventilation tubes ('grommets') are inserted through the eardrum and left in position. The purpose of these is to ventilate the eardrum in an endeavour to prevent further build-up of fluid. These tubes remain in position for around 1 year to 18 months, when, in the vast majority of cases, they fall out spontaneously.
3. Removal of the **adenoids** is also advised by some ear, nose and throat surgeons in an attempt to free the passage of fluid down the Eustachian tube – but again this is controversial.

Improving the child's hearing with the help of **hearing aids** for a short while is also being tried. Results are promising, the children tolerating the hearing aids well.

Most children who have suffered from secretory otitis media with an associated deafness usually have normal hearing by the time they are 7 or 8 years old. This appears to be the natural history of the disease, and is apparently unrelated to the type of treatment previously given. At this time, with this satisfactory result, hearing aids will no longer be required.

One further cause of a conductive deafness is a **build-up of wax** in the external auditory meatus – the passage from the exterior down to the ear-drum. This can easily be seen with an auroscope, and removed, either by syringing or by making the hard wax more fluid with ear drops. Occasionally it is necessary to soften especially hard wax with ear drops before syringing.

THE FUTURE

There is rarely any return of the conductive deafness in later life. The usual, temporary, catarrhal deafness following a head cold will, of course, still occur, but rarely persists for any length of time.

SELF-HELP GROUP

The National Deaf Children's Society
45 Hereford Road
London W2 5AH
(Tel: 071 229 9272)

This group gives advice to parents on health and education issues, and support through local groups. There are also a number of leaflets available on many aspects of deafness, together with a quarterly magazine.

Diabetes

Alternative names

'Sugar' diabetes.

Diabetes mellitus (this is the correct name for this condition, and distinguishes it from diabetes insipidus, a condition associated with disease of the pituitary gland).

INCIDENCE

Diabetes is known world-wide and the incidence varies widely. Epidemiology of this disease has unearthed some fascinating facts. It would seem that parts of the world furthest away from the equator (either north or south) have a higher incidence of diabetes than those countries nearer the equator. For example, the number of people with this disease in France is far lower than in Finland. Even such short distances as between the south of England and the north of Scotland show a distinct difference, the incidence being twice as high in Scotland.

The average number of schoolchildren with diabetes in Britain is thought to be between 1 and 2 children in every 1000. Diabetes is rare in those under 2 years. Adolescence is the most usual time for the onset of diabetes, and in this age group there is a slight preponderance of boys with the condition.

There are two main types of diabetes – the non-insulin-dependent type and the insulin-dependent type. Children predominantly have the insulin-dependent type, although the other type is not completely unknown. Further discussion will relate to the insulin-dependent type in children.

HISTORY

Diabetes has been known as a disease entity since 1500 BC. It was in the second century that a Turkish physician coined the name 'diabetes' (meaning a siphon). At this time the disease was thought to be a condition arising in the kidneys, due to the large amounts of urine passed in the acute disease. It was not until the nineteenth century that diabetes was known to be a condition caused by malfunction of the pancreas. Dietary measures were the sole treatment available at this time.

In 1922, Drs Banting and Best discovered that insulin could be used to successfully treat diabetes.

H.G. Wells was a well-known literary sufferer from diabetes. He, and Dr Lawrence, were instrumental in founding the British Diabetic Association.

CAUSATION

Diabetes is due to special cells – to be found in the islets of Langerhans within the pancreas – failing to produce insulin in adequate amounts. Insulin is a substance that is vital to the proper metabolism of sugars in the body. It is this incomplete – or inadequate – metabolism of sugars that gives rise to the symptoms of diabetes.

The precise mechanism by which diabetes occurs is not completely understood. But there are three distinct groups of factors that have a bearing on the onset of the disease, as follows.

1. **Genetic:** whilst diabetes is not a truly inherited disease, there are strong family links in the incidence. This is especially so for the insulin-dependent type of diabetes most usually seen in children. Children with two diabetic parents run a greater risk of developing the disease than children who either have only one parent with the disease or no positive family history of the condition. A child with two diabetic parents and a brother or sister with the disease stands a 50% chance of also suffering from diabetes. Recent genetic studies have shown a strong association between the development of diabetes in childhood and a particular 'marker' on chromosome 6. Factors other than genetic ones will then determine whether or not the full-blown disease occurs.

2. **Environmental** causes appear to exert some effect on the onset of diabetes. These causes only appear to affect people who already have some genetic predisposition. The commonest of these environmental causes appears to be infection of one kind or another. A viral infection with the Coxsackie B or mumps virus seems especially likely to be a predisposing factor. As most of these types of infections occur during the autumn and winter months, this would relate to the higher incidence during these times of the year. Other environmental factors, such as chemical toxins and nutritional aspects, may also have a bearing on the onset of diabetes in people with a predisposition.

3. **Immune mechanisms** have received much interest in recent years as possible causative factors in the onset of diabetes. It is known that there

is a strong association between insulin-dependent diabetes and auto-immune disease of the endocrine glands such as the thyroid and adrenal glands. Further research into this aspect has important implications for both prevention and treatment of diabetes.

Diabetes is a wide-ranging disorder with many factors to be taken into account when the causation is debated. All people with diabetes probably have a genetic predisposition (known or unknown in the family tree).

CHARACTERISTICS

Diabetes in 90% of children with the disease has an acute onset – usually with a history of various signs and symptoms of less than a month. In the remaining 10% the same symptoms occur, but in a milder form over a longer period of time.

Symptoms and signs of diabetes in a child include the following.

- Frequent passage of **urine**: this may show itself in some children as a return to bed-wetting (or even daytime wetting) after a period of complete bladder control. (It is therefore vital that all children with enuresis should have the urine tested for glucose – see elsewhere in the book.)
- An increasing **thirst**: as the frequency of the passage of urine increases, so will the child's thirst increase.
- **Weight loss**: this loss can occur rapidly in an acute onset of diabetes, the child losing many grams in a week or two.
- **Loss of energy**, together with **lethargy** and **exhaustion**, will soon become obvious. At this stage the child is seriously ill.
- **Irritation** around the vulval region in girls or the penis in boys can occur due to the passage of sugar-loaded urine.
- Occasionally, **abdominal pain** and **vomiting** may be added symptoms. Under these circumstances diagnosis can be delayed if a sample of urine is not tested for glucose, the pain and sickness being thought to be due to a gastrointestinal upset. This type of onset occurs more often in younger children.
- In a severe case of diabetes, the **breath** will have a distinctive sweet smell – similar to that of acetone or pear-drops.
- In a serious undiagnosed case the result can be **coma** and death unless correct and immediate treatment is given.

INVESTIGATIONS

Urine testing for glucose is vital for the early diagnosis of diabetes. If glycosuria is found, there should be an immediate referral to hospital. In a severe case, the urine will also show a positive result when tested for ketones. These substances will be being secreted due to the breakdown of bodily tissues, and account for the sweet smell on the breath of an undiagnosed diabetic.

Blood tests for glucose will confirm a high level of sugar in the blood. Levels of this blood sugar will need to be done frequently during the subsequent treatment of diabetes.

MANAGEMENT

Treatment for **acute onset** of diabetes is an emergency. Rapid hospital admission is necessary for treatment of the seriously ill child. Intravenous fluids and insulin are the basis of this very specialized treatment regime.

A child with a slower and less acute onset will still need to be admitted to hospital once the diagnosis is made in order to set up the regime for the future treatment of diabetes. (In a very few centres – Leicester in England and Tel Aviv in Israel – sufficient expertise is available in the community to treat children at this stage of their illness at home. Continuous ongoing monitoring is vital during these first few days following diagnosis. Usually in these centres this is provided by specially trained nurses.)

About one week in hospital is usually necessary to stabilize the diabetes on the dosage of insulin necessary for the child's needs. Much care needs to be taken to be sure that the parents fully understand the basic principles behind the twin methods of the control of their child's diabetes – **diet** and **insulin**.

For good control of the diabetes, the **diet** must be tailored to meet the needs of each individual child without causing too much difficulty in adhering to the new pattern of eating. It is necessary to avoid children feeling unusual amongst their peers, as failure to understand this will cause problems of sticking to the diet.

It is the intake of carbohydrate-containing foods that needs to be controlled in a diabetic's diet. Regular measured amounts of this type of food must be eaten. This basically means a helping of carbohydrate as follows: breakfast, mid-morning snack, lunchtime, mid-afternoon snack, supper, snack at bedtime.

A system of 'exchange' foods is worked out – each unit of 'exchange' food is equal to 10 g of carbohydrate. This system allows for a wide variety of foods to be eaten, so ensuring that a balanced diet is achieved. The carbohydrate portion of the diet should consist of starchy, high-fibre foods rather than the more quickly absorbed refined sugary foods. These starchy foods are absorbed more slowly over a longer period of time, so giving better control of the diabetes. Such foods include wholemeal bread and cereals, leguminous and green vegetables and fruits of all kinds.

The amount of carbohydrate taken in any one day should be – as a rough guide – 100 g for a 1-year-old child plus an extra 10 g daily for each added year. So, for example, a 10-year-old child will need 190 g of carbohydrate every day.

Each individual child will need to have a daily diet worked out initially by a dietician, together with a list of 'exchangeable' foods. It is surprising how quickly both children and parents become adept at estimating the amount of carbohydrate foods which make up a 10 g portion.

Adolescence is a particular time when dietary control can cause problems. Adolescents are not the most sensible of eaters at the best of times, and diabetic youngsters are no exception. Add to these problems the stress of examinations, career choices and boy/girlfriend problems and this time of life can be seen to be fraught with difficulties of control. At this time, too, the child will be moving on from the paediatric diabetic clinic to the adult diabetic clinic. All these changes need sensitive handling.

Insulin is needed for the control of the vast majority of diabetic children. Control with diet alone is very rarely achievable in childhood.

The ideal to achieve is a regime of insulin which matches the output of insulin in a normal child. This is virtually impossible, but every individual child must be balanced on the dose of insulin that matches his or her physiology as closely as possible.

Insulin usually needs to be injected twice a day, although some children may be able to manage on just one daily injection. There are short, intermediate and long-acting insulins available which can be 'mixed and matched' to suit the child's individual needs. This dosage will need to be carefully monitored by the diabetic clinic once the child has left hospital.

During the **initial** stay in hospital, both parents and child must be fully **informed** about the nature of the disease and its control. The actual physical process of injecting the insulin must also be taught. Most children over the age of 8 or 9 years will eventually be able to give their own injections. But parents must always make sure that this is done regularly and competently.

The child's **school** must be informed of the child's diabetes. Teachers should also be told of the action to take if a hypoglycaemic (see below) attack should occur in school. Such individual needs as, for example, the giving of some readily absorbed glucose before a period of strenuous activity must be fully understood – and implemented – by the staff.

Emotional support will be needed in the early days following diagnosis, especially if the child is the first member of the family to suffer from the disease. Parents must understand that diabetes is a life-long condition for which, at present, there is no cure. They must equally understand that a full, exciting life can still be led by their child if control of the diabetes is strictly maintained.

Careers for children with diabetes will need to be carefully chosen. The risk of hypoglycaemic attacks in insulin-dependent diabetes is a very real one, and diabetic people are not usually accepted for the armed forces, police or fire brigade because of this. Individual employers usually have their own rules regarding the type of work most suitable for diabetic people within their own organizations.

Hobbies, too, will need to be more carefully chosen than for the non-diabetic child. Any activity in which hypoglycaemia could put the child or the child's companions at risk should not be recommended.

Travel may present problems in control. For example, time changes when travelling long distances can cause difficulties in the timing of injections. More – or less! – activity on holidays can also make differences in the dosage of insulin necessary.

When the child reaches the age of learning to **drive**, the Driver and Vehicle Licensing Authority, in Britain, must be informed of the diabetic condition. Driving licences are granted on a 3-yearly basis, and a satisfactory medical report is needed before they can be reissued. There is rarely any problem with this. (All drivers should, of course, have a supply of sugar in the car at all times to counteract any hypoglycaemia.)

COMPLICATIONS

Hypoglycaemia

Hypoglycaemia (low blood sugar) is an ever-present complication for anyone on regular insulin. Due to a variety of factors (too little breakfast after having an insulin injection, or too much exercise combined with insufficient food, to quote just two examples) the ratio of insulin to carboyhydrate is upset. Too much insulin or too little carbohydrate will mean that the blood sugar becomes too low and this will give rise to certain specific symptoms:

* dizziness and faintness;
* nausea;
* headache;
* irritability;
* and eventually unconsciousness.

Younger children will be unable to verbalize exactly just how they are feeling, and may just say they feel 'odd' or 'funny'. Parents and teachers will get to know what is the matter under these circumstances and give appropriate treatment. Obviously, if a child has become unconscious, a 999 call will be necessary.

Treatment is quick and easy in the early stages of a hypoglycaemic attack. A sweetened drink or a lump of sugar will return the child to normal.

Most hospitals will allow a child to become hypoglycaemic deliberately whilst the parents are present so that the symptoms can be recognized, and so dealt with quickly.

Later complications

Vision can be affected by diabetes, due to the effect the disease has on the small blood vessels of the body.

Due to a similar effect on blood vessels, the **kidneys** can also be affected, as can other parts of the vascular system.

These later complications are rarely seen in childhood. Nevertheless it is of importance that good control of the disease is maintained throughout childhood in order to keep these latter complications to a minimum.

Special care needs to be taken during **pregnancy** with the control of the mother's diabetes. The baby will also need extra supervision after birth.

THE FUTURE

Diabetes is a life-long disease and at present can only be controlled and not cured. Research is proceeding along a number of lines, such as a search for possible preventable environmental triggers, the newer types of insulin and the introduction of less toxic immunosuppressant drugs which will allow pancreative –or islet cell – transplantation.

SELF-HELP GROUP

British Diabetic Association
10 Queen Anne Street
London W1M 0BD
(Tel. 071 323 1531)

This group has much useful literature available, together with a diet information service and educational and activity holidays arranged. Research into diabetes is also promoted and funded.

Diphtheria

INCIDENCE

Diphtheria has been an almost unknown infection in western countries for several decades. With the advent of routine immunization of all children against this infection from the late 1940s, the incidence has fallen dramatically. From a figure of around 45 000 a year, with over 2000 deaths, in the late 1940s, the number of cases of diphtheria between the years 1986 and 1991 was 13, with no deaths.

The picture is different, however, in many other countries of the world. In developing countries, diphtheria still takes a tragic toll of young life in terms of both illness and death. However, within the last year or so, there have been reports of many thousands of cases of diphtheria in Russia and eastern European countries. This emphasizes that continual vigilance is still necessary for the control of this infection.

HISTORY

The bacterium causing diphtheria was discovered by a Dr Klebs in 1881. Soon after this date the toxin produced by the bacterium was described, and in 1894 an antiserum was developed. A further 20 years saw the advent of a preparation which could be used to actively immunize against infection.

Dr Schick developed, in 1913, a specific skin test by which individuals immune to the effects of the bacterium could be recognized. This test is rarely used today, but at times can still be of value in determining the immune state of people working in occupations where they may come into contact with the diphtheria bacillus in the course of their work.

CAUSATION

Diphtheria is caused by a bacterium. There are three different strains of this bacterium, each giving rise to illness of differing severity.

The diphtheria bacillus produces a powerful toxin which is the cause of many of the generalized symptoms of the illness. It is also this toxin that is responsible for the serious effects seen in the heart and the nervous system.

Diphtheria is spread from person to person by droplet infection, or from clothing contaminated by the organism. Although readily destroyed by heat and antiseptic preparations, diphtheria bacteria can survive for several weeks in both milk and water. A further way of spread of this organism is from the 'carrier' state, in which some healthy people harbour the organism while suffering no ill-effects themselves.

The incubation period of the disease is between 2 and 7 days.

CHARACTERISTICS

The severity of the infection depends on the strain of the infecting organism, the 'gravis' strain producing the most severe symptoms. At times the infection can be so mild as to pass undiagnosed, the symptoms being thought to be those of a relatively mild respiratory infection. This, of course, poses problems relating to the spread of the disease – especially amongst unimmunized children.

In more severe cases the infection will begin with the following generalized symptoms.

- **Fever**: this does not usually reach as high a level as with a throat infection with streptococcal bacteria, but can reach 39.5°C. It is important that the two infections are differentiated.
- **Headache** and general **malaise**.
- **Sore throat**: this is not such an overwhelmingly unpleasant symptom as the sore throat found in an infection with streptococcal bacteria, but is nevertheless not comfortable. It is later in the course of the illness that the diphtheretic **membrane** appears in some part of the throat. This is a greyish membrane adherent to the underlying tissues which on removal leaves the under-surface raw. The danger of this membrane is that it can spread over the whole throat and soft palate – and maybe further down the respiratory tree into the larynx and bronchi – and effectively exclude the passage of air to the lungs.

As the disease progresses with the production of the specific toxin, the child's general condition deteriorates. The heart muscle can become involved, giving rise to a **weak, irregular pulse**. The **blood pressure** will fall and the child will be gravely ill.

In addition, the nervous system can become involved.

(These latter serious effects will be seen in an infection with the most serious strain of the diphtheria bacillus in a child who is not immunized against the disease.)

INVESTIGATIONS

Throat swabs – if possible taken from beneath the membrane – will confirm (or otherwise) the diagnosis of diphtheria.

MANAGEMENT

Anti-toxin: it is vital that anti-toxin – by injection – is given as soon as possible, before the toxin has become fixed in the tissues. Once this has occurred, the opportunity to counteract its effects is lost. If anti-toxin is given on the first day of the illness, full recovery is the usual result.

Antibiotics – penicillin or erythromycin – will also be necessary to ensure that a 'carrier' state does not result.

Tracheotomy may be necessary in severe cases where the diphtheretic membrane is causing obstruction to breathing.

Skilled **nursing care** in hospital is necessary for children with a severe infection of diphtheria. (It is also important to remember that added complications – see below – in the heart and nervous system can occur some weeks after the initial symptoms of diphtheria are obvious.)

COMPLICATIONS

Heart: this vital organ can be affected by the toxin produced by the diphtheria bacillus. The heart muscle itself is weakened, and so is unable to perform adequately its function of pumping the blood around the body. It is this direct effect on the heart muscle that causes the irregular heart beat, weak pulse, low blood pressure and other symptoms of heart failure in a severe case of diphtheria.

Respiration can be severely affected if the membrane extends down into the larynx. If this occurs the sufferer will have a hoarse voice and a 'brassy' cough. Breathing will be extremely difficult and the child will be restless and anxious.

Secondary infection of the respiratory tract by other organisms can occur, giving rise to **bronchopneumonia**.

The **nervous system** can also be affected by diphtheria bacteria. Weakness and/or paralysis of any muscle, or group of muscles, of the body can occur. For example the muscles of the eye can be involved, giving rise to a squint, or the arms or legs can become paralysed.

These effects occur late in the illness – often many weeks after the involvement of the throat.

PREVENTION

Diphtheria is entirely preventable by immunization, as is verified by the dramatic fall in the incidence of the disease following mass immunization.

In Western countries immunization against diphtheria is a stable part of the routine babyhood immunization schedules. In Britain, diphtheria is part of the 'triple' immunization offered to all babies at 2, 3 and 4 months of age. A 'booster' dose is given at school entry.

Children who are known to have been in close contact with a case of diphtheria should receive a further injection of vaccine. Close family contacts should also be given a 7-day course of erythromycin to ensure that a 'carrier' state does not result.

THE FUTURE

With early adequate treatment, there are no subsequent effects following an attack of diphtheria – once, of course, the period of time for the late manifestations of the disease has passed. It is if the toxin has severely damaged the heart muscle that late effects in this system of the body can be seen.

Eczema

Alternative names

Atopic dermatitis.
Infantile eczema.

INCIDENCE

There are a number of types of eczema, varying in classification. 'Contact' eczema or dermatitis is a good example of an eczematous condition in which there is a definite correlation between cause and subsequent effect. An example of this is the eczema which can occur in some people on contact with certain metals – the nickel used in jewellery, scissors or cooking utensils – or the rubber preservative chemicals used in rubber gloves.

Eczema affects around 5% of people, and the vast majority of these show signs of the condition in childhood, often below the age of 6 months. Boys and girls are equally liable to be affected.

Hay-fever, asthma and eczema are allergic conditions which frequently occur in different members of the same family. Seventy per cent of children with eczema have other family members with one or other of these allergic manifestations.

'Atopic' eczema – the type of eczema which will be further discussed – is a genetically determined skin condition in which specific antibodies can be demonstrated in the blood. Often the 'triggering' factor initiating the rash proves difficult, or impossible, to find.

HISTORY

Eczema has been known since antiquity. The word 'eczema' is derived from the Greek word meaning 'to boil out' – a good descriptive term for the red, bubbling nature of the eczema rash.

CAUSATION

Genetic factors are certainly at work in the child with atopic eczema, and it may be possible to discover certain foods or conditions which make the rash worse. For example, some babies have an, often temporary, allergy to cow's milk or they are allergic to some particular material found in clothing – wool is often a culprit here. These triggering factors have to be discovered by trial and error.

CHARACTERISTICS

The baby/child with eczema will usually have a **dry skin**, which will be in evidence from the earliest days of life.

The typical **rash** of eczema – patches of reddened skin with small blistery spots – will be extremely **irritating**. The baby will scratch, so making the skin further inflamed and the discomfort even worse.

Eczema typically occurs on the baby's **face**, and in the **knee and elbow creases**. In severe cases much of the body can be covered with the rash.

Some children experience a worsening of their rash during **cold weather**, whilst other sufferers find the rash worst during **hot, humid conditions**. This variability in manifestations of the rash can make management difficult. Each child has to be treated individually.

Improvement in the rash is occasionally seen in children between the ages of **2 and 4 years**. Unfortunately, this remission of symptoms is often short-lived, and the eczema returns again during the school-age years.

MANAGEMENT

Children with eczema have – and always will have – a very dry skin. **Emollient (greasy) creams**, applied twice every day, reduce this dryness and minimize the outbreaks of severe eczema. When the worst of the rash is absent, it is important to continue with creams to reduce the dryness.

Soap and **bubble bath** have the effects of drying the skin even further, and so should be avoided for children with a dry skin. Bath oil should be substituted for other bath-time additives, and a minimum of – preferably unperfumed – soap should be used. Moisturizers should always be applied after a bath.

Wool is a particularly frequent irritant to children with atopic eczema. (The distinction here between atopic and contact eczema is blurred.) Most eczema sufferers will react badly to even a minimum of wool in their clothing. Sometimes **acrylic** cloth can also have deleterious effects. Cotton and cotton/polyester fabrics are the most suitable ones to be worn next to the skin in eczema sufferers. (It must also be remembered that carpets and other furnishing materials can contain a certain percentage of wool. Crawling babies with an eczematous tendency can suffer from the effects of such household furnishings.)

In comparatively rare circumstances, certain **foods** can cause a worsening of eczema. This must be distinguished from the rapid allergic reaction, known as urticaria, which arises when the specific food touches the child's mouth.

Avoidance of all of the above factors which have been shown to worsen the eczema is important in the ongoing care of a child with eczema. Treatment of an acute relapse includes the following.

- A **steroid cream**, applied only to the parts of the skin which have eczematous patches, will help all but the most resistant eczema. These creams should be applied three times daily for a short time. Parents can become concerned regarding the use of steroid creams on their children's skins. They can be reassured that there is no danger of overuse as long as the treatment is not continued for an indefinite period.
- In very severe cases, particularly in young babies where control of scratching is a major problem, **wet dressings** are of value. A greasy cream is applied all over the child's body, with a steroid cream applied to the worst of the eczematous patches. Damped cotton material is then bandaged on over these creams. This treatment needs to be done three times daily, and may need a short stay in hospital. This treatment has the effect of moisturizing the skin which aids the action of the steroid creams. The irritation is reduced and, being completely bandaged, the baby cannot get at the rash to scratch his or her skin.
- If the eczema has become **infected** due to repeated scratching, **antibiotics** taken by mouth will be needed to control this. An antibiotic/steroid cream can also usefully be applied to the rash.
- Sedation at night – when the irritation is often at its worst – with an antihistamine can also help to reduce the amount of excoriation of the skin.

Eczema is a miserable, long-term problem. Parents and children will need much **support** (preferably from the same doctor who knows the ups and downs of the individual child's eczema) to cope with the inevitable remissions which occur. It is important to emphasize that acute flare-ups can be reduced to a minimum by constant adherence to methods of reducing the dryness of the child's skin and avoidance of known triggering factors.

School days can be unhappy for eczema sufferers if teachers and pupils are not informed of the recurrent and, of particular importance, the non-infectious nature of the condition. There is no sadder sight than a child with eczema being left out of activities due to an exacerbation of the rash, and the lack of understanding of the child's peers.

THE FUTURE

Eczema will be a constant companion to many of the childhood sufferers throughout life. When the time comes to choose a career, attention must be paid to avoiding choices which could worsen the possibility of an acute exacerbation of the eczema. Work with chemicals of any kind should be avoided, for example, and hairdressing, where there is much contact with soap products and various chemicals, is not a sensible choice.

SELF-HELP GROUPS

National Eczema Society
4 Tavistock Place
London WC1H 9RA
(Tel. 071 388 4097)

has information packs available on many aspects of life with eczema, as well as various support groups. Joint holiday programmes are also available, in conjunction with the National Asthma Campaign, for youngsters with severe eczema.

SIMILAR SKIN RASHES

There are a number of other forms of skin rash which are very similar to eczema and which are worthy of mention, as confusion is common.

Discoid eczema

As the name implies, this is a true form of eczema, but appears in very specific round patches. In younger children the upper arms and shoulders are the most frequently affected parts of the body. These patches can become very large, with a moist surface. They can be difficult at times to distinguish from impetigo.

Steroid creams and moisturizing ointments are the best forms of treatment.

Seborrhoeic dermatitis

This condition is frequently confused with eczema, especially in younger children and babies. The common 'cradle-cap' seen in children under 1 year of age is an example of sebhorrhoeic dermatitis. In this condition the front of the child's hair is covered in a yellowish crust, even extending to the eyebrows at times, which, when gently removed, is seen to have a red, angry base. Other parts of the body can also be affected, such as the armpits, round chubby necks and the groin.

Unlike eczema, this rash does not itch, and so secondary infection is not a problem. Treatment for cradle-cap is to apply warm olive oil to the thick scales as a softening process before applying a specific cream to remove the surface skin. In other parts of the body a weak steroid cream is the better form of treatment. An anti-seborrhoeic shampoo can also be of value.

Seborrhoeic dermatitis is unusual in later childhood, but can return in adult life.

Enuresis

Alternative name

Bed-wetting.

INCIDENCE

All young babies are wet at night as well as during the day. By 3 years of age, many children are dry by day and a few are also dry at night.

By 5 years of age, most children have ceased wetting the bed except, perhaps, on a few occasions when sickening for a cold or some other infection, for example. There are, however, around 10% of children who are still enuretic at night on a regular basis. This figure falls to 1% or less by the time adolescence is reached.

Boys tend to take longer to achieve night-time bladder control than do girls.

CAUSATION

For convenience, enuresis is divided into primary and secondary enuresis. Primary enuresis is said to occur when a child has never been dry at night apart from, possibly, a few odd occasions. Secondary enuresis is when a child who has previously been dry at night starts wetting again.

Primary enuresis may be caused by a physical abnormality in the renal tract, or due to a neurological cause. It is important to exclude any such physical abnormality before commencing treatment for the enuresis.

Developmental delay in this particular aspect of growing up may be the sole cause of the problem. This is by far the commonest cause of primary enuresis.

Secondary enuresis is also common. There can frequently be found a precipitating cause for the renewed onset of bed-wetting after, perhaps, many months of dry beds. The arrival of a new baby, starting school, marital disharmony or the death of a grandparent are all examples of stressful events in a child's life. In one who has only precarious bladder control, any of these events can be a precipitating factor in the occurrence, or onset, of wet beds.

Social deprivation and low intelligence can also be possible factors in both forms of enuresis.

CHARACTERISTICS

These are obvious, and entail the child waking in the morning to find urine has been passed in the bed with no knowledge that this has happened. It is important that parents and child-carers understand that this is not a purposeful act on the part of the child just to be difficult. He or she is genuinely unaware that the bed is wet when waking initially in the morning. So punishment has absolutely no part to play in the treatment of enuresis.

Sometimes other factors noted in the child's **behaviour** are associated with the enuresis. For example, difficulties at school or temper tantrums can be signs that the child is under stress.

Daytime wetting is also found in some children with night-time enuresis. This can point to some abnormality in the renal tract or to a urinary infection. Both these conditions must be excluded before treatment of the enuresis is begun.

Enuresis also has a definite **familial pattern**. Parents of children with enuresis frequently admit to being late in achieving bladder control themselves. If this is the case, they will have a more sympathetic outlook on the problem than those parents who had no such bladder difficulties themselves when young.

INVESTIGATIONS

The **history** of the time of onset, duration and any treatment already tried must first of all be carefully ascertained.

Following this, all children with enuresis should have a **clinical examination** with special reference to the urinary tract and any possible neurological problems. Included in this examination, for example, must be palpation of the abdomen to be sure that the kidneys are not enlarged.

If anything abnormal is discovered, an ultrasound examination is done. This will confirm the clinical findings.

The reflexes (e.g. knee and ankle jerks) will give information on the normal, or otherwise, working of the nervous system which is closely connected with bladder control.

A **sample of urine** must be sent to the laboratory to exclude any possible infection in the urinary tract which could have a bearing on the enuretic problem. A 'dipstick' test of a sample of urine should also be done to exclude glycosuria (passing of excess sugar in the urine).

Enuresis is rarely – if ever – the sole sign of diabetes in a child but this, too, should be excluded as a possible cause for the bed-wetting.

MANAGEMENT

In all but around 1% of the 10% of children who are still wetting the bed at the age of 5 years, the problem will eventually resolve itself within a few years without any specific treatment. But much distress, to both mother and child, can occur along the way unless help is given. There are several paths that can be followed to speed up normal developmental progress of this particular aspect of growing up. Until the age of around 5 years of age it is unwise to begin any systematic treatment. A relaxed attitude by parents, without censure for wet beds, will often result in a sudden succession of dry beds. Merely talking about the problem and learning how common it is can exert a magical effect on the whole family. But if such simple measures have not succeeded, there are a number of ways in which help can be given.

Star charts: by the time the enuretic child has reached the stage of having professional advice, this form of help – in one form or another – has often already been tried. Basically the idea behind such charts is to encourage children to 'log' for themselves successful dry nights.

Enuresis clinics, which are run by some general practitioners and/or local authorities, will have available standard charts of various kinds. These all put emphasis on success rather than failure. In many cases this ritual, initiated by someone outside the immediate family, can be successful within a few weeks. If there is no, or little, success with this simple method after 3–4 months, other forms of treatment are indicated.

Lifting the child from sleep when parents go to bed and taking the child to the lavatory can be tried along with the star chart. Again, if no success is gained by this, or the child becomes distressed by being woken, this should be stopped.

The **alarm** is probably one of the most well-known and advertised treatments for enuresis. It consists of a detector pad, powered by a battery, on which the child lies, separated by a sheet. If urine is passed through the sheet onto this pad the circuit is completed and the alarm sounds. There are a number of different types of alarm available. Some result in a loud buzzing noise when the circuit is completed (often waking the whole household!) whilst others only make a minimal sound from a device pinned to the child's night-clothes.

It is important that both mother and child should be shown together how to arrange, and test, the alarm. Failure to take time to do this can result in much disillusionment for both parent and child if the alarm fails to sound if urine has been passed in the night. It is important that follow-up, by someone skilled in the use of these alarms, is done on a regular basis. Minor adjustments, or repairs to the alarm, can make all the difference between success and failure. Alarms can be borrowed in some parts of the country from surgeries or local authority clinics. They can also be purchased from pharmacists by mail order.

If there has been no success with the alarm after 3 or 4 months of use, it is advisable to cease using this method for 6 months or so, and then to try again.

Success rates with the alarm are good – around 80% – if it is used properly and with a positive attitude.

Regular patterns of emptying the bladder during the day should be encouraged.

Emotional stress of any kind should be talked through with both parent and child. The causes of stress can be wide-ranging, from the trivial and easily corrected to the serious and potentially difficult to alter. If there are deep-seated problems, the help of a psychiatrist may be needed.

Goal-setting: it may be helpful to suggest to the child a goal for becoming dry such as, for example, a weekend camp, or a visit to grandparents which includes an overnight stay. Such ruses, however, should be used with caution, as failure will cause further disillusionment.

There are two other forms of treatment which are sometimes suggested, both of which have limited success and are inadvisable.

Restriction of fluids during the day only results in a thirsty child and a more irritable bladder due to concentrated urine. Obviously a large drink just before bedtime is not a sensible idea, but the child should be allowed to drink as much as desired during the day.

Tricyclic antidepressants have an initial success, but relapse almost invariably occurs once the medication has been stopped.

THE FUTURE

Once dry beds have been achieved for a period of several weeks, relapse rarely occurs – except perhaps temporarily at the onset of some infection.

The 1% of children who persist with enuresis into adolescence have difficult problems to overcome. All efforts must be made to ensure that no physical or emotional problems have been missed as a cause for the continuation of enuresis.

Epilepsy

Alternative names

The 'falling sickness'.
Fits.
Convulsions.
Seizures.
(These three latter names are frequently used synonymously when
discussing the manifestations due to epilepsy. This will
apply here.)

INCIDENCE

Epilepsy can be defined as 'a recurrent sudden electrical discharge in the brain occurring in the absence of fever'. It is this abnormal discharge that produces the typical signs and symptoms of an epileptic seizure. The type of effects seen will depend on which part of the brain is affected. There can be generalized seizures affecting the whole body, and partial seizures affecting only certain parts or senses.

In school-aged children, the incidence of epilepsy is between 4 and 9 children for every 1000. (In pre-school children, febrile convulsions – seen only in the under-5's – have a different incidence, aetiology and course. These convulsions are the direct result of a sudden rise in temperature in the immature brain, and are grown out of by the fifth birthday.) The incidence of febrile convulsions is around 3% of all pre-school children.

There are a number of conditions which, at first sight, can closely resemble epilepsy. For example, breath-holding attacks and acute labyrinthitis can closely mimic an epileptic attack. These conditions must be carefully excluded before a diagnosis of epilepsy is made, with all the treatment and restrictions that such a diagnosis can imply.

Epilepsy is known in all countries of the world, and affects both sexes.

HISTORY

Epilepsy has been described since Biblical times, and, for many years, has unjustly stigmatized sufferers from this disorder. People suffering from epilepsy have frequently been described as 'devil-possessed' or 'mad'. Fortunately, today there is a better understanding of the cause, and the course, of this condition, together with successful drug treatments for the different types of epilepsy. But continuing further education of the public about these – often frightening to witness – episodes is still necessary.

CAUSATION

Fits can be part of the **symptomatology** of **complex syndromes**, such as, for example, the Sturge–Weber syndrome and Batten's disease. (The figure of 140 genetic disorders associated with seizures has been quoted.)

Genetic inheritance appears to have a bearing on the occurrence of primary generalized – or idiopathic – epilepsy. It is thought that the risk of the children of epilepsy sufferers having the disorder is in the region of around 8%.

Developmental abnormalities in the structure of the brain can be the basis of the epilepsy. Some children who show generalized developmental delay can also have seizures as part of the general picture.

Chemical imbalance in the body can give rise to fits under certain conditions. For example, low calcium or magnesium levels can cause this problem, particularly in newborn babies, as can, under certain circumstances, low blood sugar. Fits due to these factors, however, cannot be classed as true epilepsy, as once the body physiology has been returned to normal, the abnormal electrical activity will cease.

Seizures can also be a long-term complication following a severe **head injury**.

Infections, both those occurring prenatally such as toxoplasmosis or infection with the cytomegalovirus, and those occurring later in childhood, can be a factor. Such serious infections as meningitis, septicaemia or encephalitis can leave the child with recurrent seizures following recovery from the acute illness.

Tumours in the brain are a further cause of the onset of seizures in a child who has no previous history of epilepsy.

It can be seen that the list of possible causes of fits is almost as long as the types of fits themselves. So great care must be taken to attempt to determine a treatable cause for the fits before a diagnosis of idiopathic epilepsy is made – with all its future implications for treatment and lifestyle.

CHARACTERISTICS

Generalized seizures

These can be divided into 'grand mal', 'petit mal' and myoclonic seizures.

Grand mal epilepsy occurs in about 80% of children who suffer from epilepsy. Before the fit, the child may **behave** in an unusual way or be especially **irritable** for some hours before the following occurs.

1. A sudden **loss of consciousness** in which the child will fall to the ground and become rigid. At this time breathing will cease and the child will become blue due to lack of oxygen. This is known as the **tonic phase** of a grand mal fit, and lasts around 30 seconds.
2. Following this there will be a phase – the **clonic phase** – in which the arms and legs will exhibit jerking movements. This phase is variable in length and can last several minutes. The movements will gradually cease and the child will slowly regain consciousness, having no memory of the seizure.
3. Finally the child may feel the need to **sleep** for a variable length of time, or may be **confused** or **irritable** for a while.

Frothing at the mouth can occur at the height of the fit, and incontinence of urine may also occur. (Biting of the tongue is an extremely unusual occurrence in spite of the many lurid stories that abound!)

Petit mal can be extremely difficult to diagnose. There are short periods of **altered consciousness** (10–15 seconds only) in which the child stops whatever he or she is doing and stares into space. Following these 'absences', the activity or conversation will be picked up again as if there had been no interval. (A further – descriptive – name for petit mal is 'absences'.)

These absences can occur many times during the day. Often the only clue that they are occurring is a fall-off in the child's school performance. Due to the frequent absences much can be missed over the course of a day's schooling. If this possibility is remembered, the child can be observed carefully and the attacks noted.

There are no involuntary movements or incontinence during these attacks of petit mal.

Myoclonic epilepsy most commonly occurs in children who have developmental delay, often due to underlying brain damage. The attacks are brief and may only consist of **jerking movements** of arms, body and/or legs. Occasionally only the head is involved in the jerky movement. The child may fall to the floor, but will recover quickly. (The Lennox–Gastaut syndrome – a specialized form of childhood epilepsy – commonly has myoclonic epilepsy as part of its symptomatology.)

Partial seizures

There are two main types of partial epileptic seizures. These arise due to abnormal electrical discharges in specific parts of the brain.

Rolandic epilepsy (or **benign partial epilepsy of childhood**) occurs between the ages of 3 and 12 years. Symptoms occur most frequently at night, or during the period between sleeping and waking. This timing can make diagnosis difficult.

The child is conscious throughout the whole attack. The child is often unable to speak, but will point to the side of the face, obviously trying to convey the unusual feelings that are occurring. During recovery, this area of the face may twitch. The whole episode is over within a couple of minutes.

Occasionally, unusual sensations of swelling or shrinking of an arm or one side of the face can be described afterwards by an articulate child.

The electroencephalogram (EEG) in this type of epilepsy shows a very typical diagnostic pattern. Fortunately this benign type of epilepsy disappears completely around the age of 12–13 years, never to reappear. The abnormal EEG tracing gradually returns to normal. Treatment is rarely necessary, but specific drugs will stop the attacks if they are occurring too frequently or the child is unduly distressed by them.

Temporal lobe epilepsy is associated with a number of bizarre symptoms. The child may have specific **hallucinations** of a visual, auditory or olfactory nature. (A splendid old black and white film had as a main character someone who could smell fried onions as a prelude to his temporal lobe seizure!)

Alternatively the sufferer may have sudden explosive attacks of rage or intense fear. Objective signs, such as flushing of the face, dilations of the pupils of the eyes or perspiration, can also occur during an attack.

These occurrences are sometimes followed by a typical grand mal attack. Following the seizure the child feels confused and will need to sleep for an hour or more, although there is no definite memory of the attack.

The causes of these attacks are due to a number of possible factors, ranging from a previous severe infection, through a previous lack of oxygen causing damage to a specific part of the brain to a cerebral tumour.

INVESTIGATIONS

A careful **history** of the attacks is the most important factor in the diagnosis of any form of epilepsy. The sequence of events as well as what actually happened – as described by a witness – will give clues as to whether the attack was epileptic or not.

Tests for **chemical imbalances** must be done on a sample of blood to exclude such conditions as diabetes or kidney failure, for example.

An **EEG** will show up any abnormalities in the brain waves. Many EEG patterns are quite specific for different forms of epilepsy.

CT scans are important follow-up investigations if it is thought that there is some physical abnormality in the brain causing the seizures.

Magnetic resonance imaging may, on occasions, be necessary to demonstrate a tiny lesion that could be missed on a CT scan.

All these investigations must, however, be interpreted in conjunction with a clear account of the actual seizure.

MANAGEMENT

Drugs: the decision to start drug treatment of epilepsy can be a difficult one. Rarely, if ever, are drugs needed for a single, or even two, seizures. But when attacks interfere with a child's everyday activities, drug treatment will be necessary – for example, when there are so many 'absences' due to petit mal during a school day as to interfere with the child's ability to learn. There are a wide range of drugs which can be used to control epilepsy. Each type of epilepsy has a drug, or group of drugs, which will best be able to control the seizures. In order to determine the drug best suited to each child's individual needs, it may be necessary to try various drugs, or two in combination. The most successful drug should then be prescribed on a long-term basis. Most children will need to take the drug of choice twice each day in order to control their fits adequately. It may be necessary to change the drug regime as the child matures. Side-effects must also be noted, and regular measurement of blood levels of the drug monitored. Side-effects include giddiness, hyperactivity, headache, blurred vision and learning difficulties. These side-effects are quite specific to each drug.

Schooling: children with epilepsy unrelated to any other pathological condition are quite able to attend an ordinary school. Figures quoted of the normal intelligence range in children with epilepsy vary between 50% and 70%. The remainder of the children will probably have a deficit in their intellectual ability due to other problems – which in themselves, of course, have a bearing on the aetiology of their seizures.

Teaching staff should be aware of their pupil's problems, and be conversant with first aid treatment in case of a fit occurring during the school day. This latter event is, however, unlikely to occur if medication is carefully prescribed – and taken.

Some children will experience **learning difficulties** as a result of their epilepsy or associated disorders. Special schooling for these children will then be necessary.

Activities: certain activities are dangerous for children with epilepsy, as follows.

- **Swimming** must always be in the presence of an adult who, ideally, should be in sole charge of the individual child.

- **Cycling** in the open road with fast-moving traffic should not be allowed.
- **Gymnastic activities** which necessitate climbing to a height up wall-bars or ropes should be forbidden. Other exercises in the gym are beneficial and should be encouraged.

Family therapy, following the initial diagnosis, can be helpful if parents are particularly upset regarding the diagnosis. General practitioners, paediatricians, health visitors and teaching staff can all be involved in helping the family come to terms with the child's epilepsy. Full explanations of what is happening, the purpose of the treatment and how best to help the child live a happy, fulfilled life are all areas that will need to be explored.

Surgery plays a minor part in the management of epilepsy. This is restricted to helping uncontrollable epilepsy in some severely handicapped children.

THE FUTURE

Driving: a driving licence can be held by people with epilepsy provided that 2 years have elapsed without a daytime seizure – whether on medication or not.

Genetic counselling, before a pregnancy is undertaken, may be necessary for some couples who have a strong family history of epilepsy.

Work: certain modes of employment are inadvisable for people with epilepsy, such as, for example, work necessitating climbing to a height or working near to continuously moving machinery. Careers advice is helpful during the later years at school.

Cessation of seizures: it has been estimated that by adulthood between 50% and 70% of children with epilepsy will have no further seizures. This, of course, is very much dependent upon the type and cause of the epilepsy.

SELF-HELP GROUPS

British Epilepsy Association
Anstey House
40 Hanover Square
Leeds LS3 1BE
(Tel. 0532 439393)

Epilepsy Association of Scotland
48 Govan Road
Glasgow G51 1JL
(Tel. 041 427 4911).

These associations provide support and information for teachers and families. Local conferences are arranged, as are holidays for children with severe epilepsy. There are information packs for schools, as well as books, leaflets and videos on all aspects of epilepsy.

Fifth disease

'Slapped cheek syndrome.'
Erythema infectiosum.

INCIDENCE

This infection affects children between the ages of 2 and 10 years. Adults can also be affected, but this is unusual. For some unknown reason, girls are more frequently affected than boys.

Outbreaks of this condition can occur at any time of the year but are most common during the winter and the spring. This is in line with the higher incidence of many infections due to the closer proximity of children to one another during the colder months of the year.

CAUSATION

Fifth disease is caused by a virus of the parvo group. The infection is spread from child to child by droplet infection. The virus is also thought to be contracted from infected blood products such as, for example, when a child has a blood transfusion for some reason. The incubation period is variable, anything from 5 to 20 days after exposure being quoted.

CHARACTERISTICS

Frequently the first sign of the 'slapped cheek syndrome' is the typical **rash** (similar in type to that seen in rubella) which appears on the child's cheeks. As the name implies, it appears as if the child has received a blow to the face. (Fifth disease must always be remembered as a possibility when there has been a previous high index of suspicion of child abuse.)

In contrast to the bright red rash on the cheeks, the area around the child's mouth is seen to be **pale**. (A similar phenomenon is seen in scarlet fever. This latter infection is, however, a far more serious and severe disease and the two infections are distinguished by the more generalized and serious constitutional upset seen in scarlet fever.) In 2 or 3 days the rash extends to the chest and limbs. This lasts for a week or two and then gradually fades, but can be seen to return for a further couple of weeks on the child having a hot bath. This rash can be mildly irritating.

There may also be a **fever** associated with the illness, this usually being in evidence before the rash appears. This, as with all feverish illness, is associated with **headache** and a general feeling of **malaise** and **aching limbs**.

INVESTIGATIONS

Blood tests: the diagnosis can be confirmed by a specialized laboratory test on a sample of blood. This is rarely performed in an uncomplicated case of fifth disease, but may be necessary if any of the rare complications occur.

MANAGEMENT

As with most viral infections, there is no specific treatment, antibiotics being of no value in infections of viral origin.

Analgesics, for control of fever if present to any degree, and to relieve headache and aching limbs, should be given if necessary. Dosage must, of course, be appropriate to the age of the child. (Aspirin must not be given to children under the age of 12 years due to the link between this analgesic and Reye's syndrome.)

It is not necessary to keep a child with fifth disease away from **school** unless they are feeling too unwell due to fever and other symptoms of infection. As infection is passed on from child to child before the rash appears, staying away from school will not help to reduce the spread of the infection. Once the rash has appeared, the child is no longer infectious.

COMPLICATIONS

A mild **arthritis** can occur with the slapped cheek syndrome, usually beginning a few days before the appearance of the rash. Although this complication more commonly occurs in adults with the infection, children can also suffer. The pain associated with the arthritis tends to come and go in a fleeting fashion, and can last many weeks. The smaller joints of the body are usually affected – fingers, wrists and ankles. Analgesics may be necessary to control this pain.

There are two special groups of children who can have complications due to fifth disease.

One of these groups of children comprises those who have **thalassaemia** or **sickle cell anaemia**. Here the infection may precipitate a 'crisis' in which levels of haemoglobin fall dangerously low. Blood transfusion may be necessary for these children until the effects of the virus have worn off.

The other group of children who can suffer from complications comprises those children with a pre-existing malignancy, particularly **acute leukaemia**. Specialized treatment is necessary under these conditions.

PREVENTION

There is no immunization available against the slapped cheek syndrome.

THE FUTURE

There is no long-term disability following an attack of fifth disease. The arthritis which sometimes occurs is only temporary and does not recur later in life.

If the disease is contracted during pregnancy, miscarriage can occur, but this is not invariably so.

Gastroenteritis

INCIDENCE

Gastroenteritis is one of the commonest of childhood infections. This is so throughout the world. Whilst the incidence of this illness has fallen steadily in the west, in many developing countries gastroenteritis is still one of the major killer diseases in children. The dramatic fall in fatalities in the west due to this infection is largely the result of improved hygiene and the energetic treatment of dehydration in children with an acute attack of gastroenteritis. Outbreaks of gastroenteritis still occur, however, in nurseries and schools, and there are isolated incidents in homes throughout the country, 50% of the cases occurring in children below the age of 5 years. This is especially so in the winter months when close contact amongst children is more usual than in the summer months.

HISTORY

Diarrhoeal disease has always been a problem where large numbers of people congregate together. Cholera, dysentery and typhoid were common gastrointestinal disorders during the last century. Since this time health measures regarding purity of drinking water and disposal of sewage have transformed the picture in developed countries.

CAUSATION

Gastroenteritis can be caused by bacteria or viruses. It is thought that around 50% of all gastroenteritis attacks are caused by the rotavirus. These tiny viruses were first detected in Australia. They can be visualized under the electron microscope.

The infection is probably passed from child to child by imperfect hand-washing after visiting the lavatory, for example. It may be that infection can also be passed on by droplet infection from the respiratory tract. Many children with a diarrhoeal disease also have had a cold a few days previously. Children up the age of 6 years are particularly prone to gastroenteritis due to these viruses. After this age, the majority of children have built up an immunity to the virus and so do not suffer from symptoms of the infection.

The 'Norwalk' virus has been one of the more publicized viruses causing gastroenteritis in recent years. But there are a number of other viruses which also cause similar unpleasant symptoms.

There are also several bacteria causing gastroenteritis. The commonest of these are the E. coli, Salmonella and Shigella bacteria. The fall in gastroenteritis cases in the west is largely due to better control of these bacteria. Outbreaks of salmonella still occur, and are usually due to contaminated food. Contact tracing of these outbreaks is energetically pursued and appropriate steps taken to improve hygiene to avoid further problems.

CHARACTERISTICS

Whatever the causative organism, the clinical signs and symptoms of an acute attack of gastroenteritis are similar.

The early stages of the infection can well be non-specific. The baby or young child will be **irritable** and **crying**, and will cease to play happily. Food will be refused, and an excessive thirst may be noticed.

Within a few hours, **vomiting** will occur, especially in younger children. This will usually precede the **diarrhoea** which soon follows. (These symptoms can also, of course, occur in other conditions which need surgery – such as, for example, appendicitis and intussusception.)

Fever is variable – sometimes only a mild fever is present whilst at other times the temperature is high. This latter occurs more frequently with an infection by the rotavirus group.

INVESTIGATIONS

Usually – and fortunately! – attacks of gastroenteritis in children are short-lived and mild. In these cases, no investigation into the causative organism is necessary. But if an outbreak in a nursery or a school, for example, occurs, samples of the stools of sufferers, and their families, should be sent to the laboratory for identification of the infecting organism.

MANAGEMENT

Toddlers and older children

In **mild cases** where vomiting and frequent diarrhoea are not a serious problem, **fluids** only should be given for 24 hours. In the young child this is usually no problem, as food is the last thing he or she will wish to see or take! Plain water, or water with the addition of a teaspoon of glucose to a glass, whenever thirst is complained of, is all that is necessary for 24 hours. Following this, provided that vomiting has ceased and the diarrhoea improved, solid food can be reintroduced gradually over the next few days.

In more **severe** cases, replacement of lost fluid by one of the **commercial replacement fluids** (obtainable from pharmacists) will be necessary. Again, no solid food should be given.

Medical advice should always be sought if the diarrhoea and vomiting are severe and/or persist for longer than a few hours. This is especially important in young children. Large amounts of fluid can be lost by severe diarrhoea and vomiting and small children cannot easily replace this loss.

Hospital admission may be necessary for the small child with a severe attack of gastroenteritis because of this fluid loss. Under these circumstances, not only is the loss of fluid itself potentially dangerous, but the blood chemistry can be seriously disturbed. Skilled medical and nursing care are required in these circumstances.

Babies under 1 year

Similar treatment is necessary for small babies as for older children. But it must be remembered that tiny babies can become dehydrated very quickly and can become dangerously ill in a very short time. So medical advice must be obtained quickly for these little ones.

Kaolin, or any of the other anti-diarrhoeal agents, are of no value in childhood gastroenteritis. Antibiotics are also of no value in gastroenteritis due to a virus, but should be used in proven cases of *Salmonella* infection.

COMPLICATIONS

Dehydration, as described above, is the most immediate and serious complication. Treatment is as described, but with emphasis on early medical help for the younger child.

Sugar intolerance is a common complication following an attack of gastroenteritis. The younger the child, the more frequently does this occur. Symptoms of this appear as soon as milk is reintroduced into the diet following the initial treatment. Diarrhoea will again become a problem, with frequent, frothy, watery stools which in turn often give rise to an unpleasant nappy-rash. (It is the sugar – lactose – in the milk that causes the problem.) The basic cause of this temporary intolerance is the damage done to the lining of the intestine by the bacteria or virus causing the gastroenteritis.

Treatment is to give a lactose-free milk for a few weeks to give the intestine time to recover. After about 4–6 weeks ordinary milk should be gradually reintroduced into the diet, and usually there is no return of the diarrhoea. If there is, the process should be repeated until ordinary milk is tolerated again.

PREVENTION

It would be good to think that all attacks of gastroenteritis in children – and adults! – could be prevented. Unfortunately it is difficult to imagine this scenario, although work is proceeding towards a vaccine against the rotavirus.

Good **hygiene** in the preparation of food and instillation of regular hand-washing after visiting the lavatory and before meals are important in controlling the spread of infection.

Medical advice should be obtained sooner, rather than later, especially in the case of young babies, in order to prevent complications.

Glandular fever

Alternative names

Infectious mononucleosis.
'Kissing' disease.

INCIDENCE

Glandular fever is usually a disease affecting older children and young adolescents. But younger children are by no means immune to the condition, although children under the age of 3 years rarely suffer from the disease.

Overcrowding and poor hygiene are factors in the spread of the infection, which is passed on by close physical contact. The virus is harboured in the throat and salivary glands – often for many months after recovery from the original infection. (This is the reason for the popular name – 'kissing' disease – of glandular fever, and is the most likely form of spread during the adolescent years.) Epidemics can also occur in schools and residential homes.

There is no particular time of the year when glandular fever is more common, cases occurring throughout the seasons.

The infection is world-wide, and occurs with equal frequency in both sexes.

HISTORY

The incidence of glandular fever appears to have changed since the earlier days of the twentieth century. At this time, younger children were the most frequent sufferers, and epidemics amongst this age group were described. These are no longer seen to occur.

CAUSATION

Glandular fever is caused by a virus of the herpes group – the Epstein–Barr virus. The incubation period is thought to be between 5 and 10 days. But due to the virus remaining in the throat and salivary glands, infection can be passed on to another individual up to 12 weeks after the initial attack.

CHARACTERISTICS

Glandular fever can be notoriously difficult to diagnose clinically. This is partly because there are a number of different ways in which the infection can manifest itself. Also, signs and symptoms at times are very similar to those of other infective conditions, such as tonsillitis or influenza. Characteristically, however, glandular fever begins with **tiredness** and a general feeling of **malaise** with **headache, muscular pains, sore throat** and **fever** – all very general signs of any infectious illness. In glandular fever, however, many of the **glands in the neck** become swollen. Swelling of the **glands in the armpit and groin** soon follows.

Occasionally in children there is a transient **rash** at the onset of the disease. (If ampicillin, an antibiotic commonly used to control infections, is given to a child who has glandular fever, a severe rash can be the result.)

The **tonsils** are seen to be red and swollen (a very similar picture to that seen in an attack of tonsillitis). Swallowing can be difficult for the youngster in severe cases.

On close examination of the mouth, the **palate** is seen to have tiny haemorrhages in the early stages of the infection. This sign is specific to glandular fever, and can help to make the diagnosis clear if seen early enough in the infection.

The **spleen** is enlarged and often tender to touch. Also, the **liver** is often enlarged, and **jaundice** may be a feature.

INVESTIGATIONS

Blood tests show a specific feature with an excess in the numbers of a particular type of white cell. A specific test on the blood – the Paul Bunnell reaction – confirms the diagnosis of glandular fever, but is only positive in 60% of cases. There is a similar rapid slide test – the 'Monospot' test – which can be performed quickly in the surgery without the need to wait for laboratory results. Both these tests can be negative in the early stages of the disease – yet a further complication! – but will be positive if repeated a week later.

Other **specific laboratory tests** done on a blood sample will show changes which will help with the diagnosis.

MANAGEMENT

There is no specific treatment for an attack of glandular fever. Acyclovir – a useful drug against some viral infections under certain conditions – is of no value against infection with the Epstein–Barr virus.

Rest (not necessarily in bed), with adequate **fluids** and a light **diet**, together with **analgesics** to relieve the pain of the sore throat and headache and plenty of sympathy are all that can be done. A **throat swab** should be taken if the tonsillar involvement is severe and the glands in the neck are tender as well as swollen. At times a secondary infection with streptococcal bacteria can add to the patient's miseries. Under these circumstances, treatment with penicillin is indicated.

Most children will completely recover from an attack of glandular fever within 3 weeks. But occasionally the feelings of malaise, mild fever and lack of appetite can drag on for weeks or months. Under these conditions it is wise for a chest X-ray to be taken to exclude any further infection in the lungs.

Difficulties can arise in older children if they succumb to an attack of glandular fever at **examination times**. There is no doubt that the child will not be able to give of his or her best if they have only recently recovered from glandular fever. Most educational authorities recognize this and make the appropriate allowances.

COMPLICATIONS

Secondary bacterial infection can occur in throat or chest, as mentioned above, and must be treated with the appropriate antibiotic.

Liver involvement, giving rise to jaundice, rarely occurs in children. If, however, it does, recovery will be complete and rapid.

Occasionally there can be a **relapse**, with symptoms similar to the original attack, after a few weeks. Again, this will resolve spontaneously with a few days' rest.

PREVENTION

Sensible precautions, such as good hygiene, avoidance of overcrowding and minimal close contact with the sufferer, are all that can be suggested by way of preventative measures.

THE FUTURE

There are no long-term after-effects from glandular fever.

Hand, foot and mouth syndrome

INCIDENCE

Small outbreaks of this graphically named infection can occur amongst babies and older children. The summer months are the most likely time for the condition to occur. Adults can suffer from the disease as well as children.

HISTORY

Hand, foot and mouth disease was first recognized as a clinical entity in Toronto in 1957. An outbreak of the infection occurred with quite specific features, and was named according to the characteristics noted. (The name bears an unfortunate resemblance to the foot and mouth disease found in cattle, but has absolutely nothing to do with this.)

CAUSATION

Hand, foot and mouth disease is caused by a virus of the Coxsackie group. The virus can be isolated from the skin lesions and also from the stools of sufferers.

The incubation period for this infection is unknown.

CHARACTERISTICS

There may be a mild constitutional upset before the typical rash appears. The child may have a mild **fever**, and complain of a **headache** and a general feeling of **malaise**.

Babies may be reluctant to take their feeds, and older children be unwilling to eat, as the rash starts to make its appearance.

The **rash** is very specific and consists of small, greyish-white blistery spots with a surrounding red halo. These are found on the tongue, making this mobile organ sore. The palms of the hands and the sides of the soles of the feet are also affected. Occasionally this rash may become more widespread, and can often be seen to cover the buttocks as well. (If the rash does occur on the buttocks, confusion can arise between this condition and Henoch–Schonlein purpura – see elsewhere in the book.)

The rash lasts between 3 and 5 days, and then fades rapidly. Other symptoms, if present, then also improve rapidly and the child is restored to full health.

MANAGEMENT

General sympathetic care is all that is required for an attack of hand, foot and mouth disease. **Fluids** only for a day or two may be required if the child's mouth is sore following the appearance of the rash. Otherwise, **bland foods** will be better tolerated than spicy, highly flavoured ones until the tongue has returned to normal.

Analgesics to reduce fever and relieve headache should be given if necessary. Paracetamol compounds only should be given to children, as the use of aspirin runs the risk, in those under 12 years, of Reye's syndrome.

School-age children should remain away from **school** whilst the rash is present on their hands. As the incubation period of this infection is unknown, the time when it can be passed on is uncertain, but, as with most viral infections, the most infectious period is probably the time just before the rash appears.

COMPLICATIONS

The only complication that has been reported to occur with this infection is for the **rash to extend** all over the body. This is rare, but must be remembered when a child is seen with a rash that covers the whole of the body. The diagnosis can be made by the very obvious greyish rash that covers the palms of the hands and soles of the feet.

THE FUTURE

There are no long-term effects in later life from hand, foot and mouth disease.

Hay-fever

Alternative name

Seasonal allergic rhinitis.

INCIDENCE

It is thought that between 10% and 20% of the population suffer from hay-fever. The time of the year at which the symptoms appear is dependent upon which particular tree or flower produces the allergy in each individual person.

Springtime – March to May – when many plants come into bloom shows the highest incidence of hay-fever. Late-flowering plants such as carnations, dahlias and chrysanthemums, as well as the common stinging nettle, can all produce symptoms later in the year, from July to September. Moulds and mildews, usually at their height during warm, damp weather, can also affect some people. So whilst hay-fever (as its name implies) is at its height during the spring, certain sufferers are not immune for the rest of the year.

Hay-fever affects both sexes equally, and even young children can be affected, although most children first begin to suffer during the early school years.

West Indian children living in Britain appear to have a higher incidence of hay-fever than usual. It has also been reported that children of non-manual workers are more prone to hay-fever.

CAUSATION

Hay-fever is the third member of the allergy trio, asthma, eczema and hay-fever. The cause is an allergic reaction to the pollens of many different types of trees and grasses and to flowers of all kinds. The amount of pollen produced by just one flower is incredible – a single sorrel flower has been reported as producing 180 000 grains of pollen. In a high wind these grains can be carried for more than 10 miles! It is therefore difficult to take avoiding action from the effects of these minute grains of pollen.

Susceptibility to these allergens is often inherited. Other members of the family may not themselves be hay-fever sufferers, but may have asthma or eczema.

Symptoms, of course, are at their worst when the pollen count is high.

CHARACTERISTICS

- Profuse clear, watery **discharge** from the **nose**, often associated with sneezing.
- **Red, runny, itchy eyes**. This symptom is sometimes known by the alternative name of 'allergic conjunctivitis', and can occur without the other symptoms of hay-fever. The causative factors are similar.
- **Wheezing** and **breathlessness** can also occur with hay-fever as well as asthma. The differential diagnosis between these two conditions can at times be blurred.
- **Itching** of the **soft palate** (and also at times the **ears**, due to a common nerve supply between these two structures).

Diagnosis is based on the occurrence of these symptoms at times of the year which are specific to each sufferer.

MANAGEMENT

It is virtually impossible to avoid contact with pollen altogether. Even if this were possible, it would be hard to keep children indoors during the warm summer months. There are a number of drug treatments available which will subdue most of the symptoms of hay-fever.

- **Eye drops** of sodium cromoglycate – the same drug that is used as a prophylactic measure in asthma – are very successful in keeping the eye symptoms under control. The drops will need to be instilled, on a regular basis, four times a day. This regime needs to be strictly adhered to throughout the hay-fever season.
- **Antihistamines** (there are those available which do not cause drowsiness) are helpful for mild cases, and again should be used throughout the season.
- **Steroids** used in an inhaler are necessary for more severe cases.
- **Steroids** given in tablet form by mouth can be used in the short term for children with disabling symptoms of hay-fever. These drugs (which are not advised for long-term use) are useful to tide a teenager with severe hay-fever over a difficult examination period.

THE FUTURE

Some sufferers find their hay-fever improves as the years go by, but most children suffering from hay-fever will continue to do so throughout their lives. It is fortunate that there are drugs available to control the symptoms.

Henoch–Schonlein purpura

Alternative name

Anaphylactoid purpura.

INCIDENCE

There are no available figures for this condition, but it is not an especially common disorder. Nevertheless, when it does occur the signs and symptoms are sufficiently severe to cause alarm and – at times – difficulties in diagnosis.

Henoch–Schonlein purpura can run a protracted course, with associated implications for both care and education. Fortunately, full recovery – in a time scale ranging from 6 weeks to 1 year – is the usual outcome of this disease.

The condition is commonest amongst pre-school children, even as young as 1 year, but all age groups can be affected.

Boys are more frequently affected than girls.

HISTORY

The double-barrelled name of this disease arose due to the involvement of two doctors – Henoch and Schonlein – in the description of the condition. Henoch described the relationship of the specific rash with the gastrointestinal symptoms, whilst Schonlein placed emphasis on the relationship of the rash with the arthritic manifestations. It was later realized that both descriptions related to the one disease.

CAUSATION

The basic cause of Henoch–Schonlein purpura is unknown, but it probably results from an immune system problem.

The pathology is one of inflammation around the capillaries and small arteries (a vasculitis) in many – and varied – parts of the body, including the skin, the gastrointestinal tract and the kidneys.

There have been suggestions that the onset of the condition may be preceded by an upper respiratory tract infection, but this is not always the case.

CHARACTERISTICS

The typical **rash** is usually the first sign of the disease. This rash consists of small 'bruise-like' ('purpuric') spots around a blistery centre which, unlike a number of other rashes, does not disappear when pressed with a finger. The rash is the result of the inflammatory process around the blood vessels.

The distribution of the rash is quite distinctive, being mainly confined to the backs of the legs and the buttocks. In some children the rash may be minimal and confined to only a few spots. But if they are seen in a child who is complaining of the other typical symptoms, the diagnosis is made clear.

The rash is painless and does not itch. As fading takes place over the succeeding days the typical yellow discoloration associated with a fading bruise is seen.

Gastrointestinal tract: symptoms in this body system are often the most unpleasant ones in Henoch–Schonlein purpura. Due to the lesions – similar to the ones seen on the skin – in the intestine, bleeding occurs. This gives rise to **colicky abdominal pain** which can either be persistent or come and go intermittently. Acute abdominal pain in children is notoriously difficult to diagnose, as there are a multitude of possible causes. It is the relationship with the skin rash that provides the clue to the diagnosis of Henoch–Schonlein purpura. **Vomiting** can also occur in association with the abdominal pain. **Blood** in the motions is a common feature, although this may not be obvious to the naked eye. Laboratory testing will confirm that bleeding has occurred into the intestine.

Children with this kind of continuing abdominal pain will often become unduly **depressed** – understandably so. There is nothing quite so lowering as continuing tummy pain.

Some **joints** of the body can be affected. The child will complain of **pain** and **tenderness**, particularly on movement. This pain, as with the abdominal pain, can be intermittent and is again due to the inflammation of the small blood vessels around the affected joints.

The **kidneys** can also be specifically involved in Henoch–Schonlein purpura. This is an especially worrying aspect of this otherwise benign disease. Long-term effects can result from the involvement of the renal tract.

As with the gastrointestinal tract, there can be bleeding from the small blood vessels in the renal tract. Again, this bleeding may not be visible in the child's urine to the naked eye, but can be demonstrated by laboratory testing. Associated with this is the passage of microscopic amounts of protein in the urine, again demonstrable in the laboratory.

The timing of the renal tract involvement can be unusual, occasionally arising as late as 3 months after the appearance of the rash. So it is important that a check should be kept on the child's urine at intervals, for several months after an attack of Henoch–Schonlein purpura. (In a few – very rare – cases, the kidney involvement is a major feature of the disease, and runs a rapidly downhill course leading to fatal renal failure.)

Henoch–Schonlein purpura is a condition which can resolve completely within 6 weeks, leaving the child in complete health. There can also be remissions back into abdominal and joint pain for as long as 1 year, with a continuation of protein being excreted in the urine, showing that the kidneys are still being affected by the disease. But in the vast majority of cases, recovery is eventually complete with no long-lasting ill effects.

INVESTIGATIONS

Blood tests show few specific changes with an attack of Henoch–Schonlein purpura.

Urine testing, as mentioned, shows varying amounts of protein and/or blood according to the degree to which the kidneys are involved in the condition.

MANAGEMENT

Whilst there are no specific drugs which will produce a dramatic cure, careful management of the – sometimes very distressing – symptoms of the disease is important.

Bed rest during the period when the rash is at its height is advised. It has been found that the rash tends to worsen if the child is allowed to run around. Also, if there is obvious bleeding from the renal tract, bed rest is advisable.

Analgesics to control the pain from tender joints will give much relief. The abdominal pain can also be controlled by analgesics. In mild cases paracetamol will suffice, but children with severe abdominal pain will need stronger drugs to control this distressing symptom. Occasionally steroids will be needed to give relief.

Emotional support for both parents and child during the possibly long duration of this disease is important. Full explanations of possible causes and the probable sequence of events should be given, so that parents can cope with each new manifestation if and when it arises. The child's possible depression also needs to be discussed, and plans made to mitigate this as far as possible.

Schooling can be resumed when the rash has disappeared and pain is absent from joints. Due to the possible relapsing course of this disease, teachers should be kept advised of problems as they arise. Work may need to be sent home if the child is not up to coping with the rough and tumble of the school day. School staff should also be reassured that the condition is not infectious.

Regular **review of kidney function** together with blood pressure measurements should be done until all signs of protein in the urine are absent.

COMPLICATIONS

The important complication of continuing renal involvement must always be borne in mind. **Hypertension** (high blood pressure) can result from severe involvement of the kidneys. If this occurs, it should be treated to avoid further problems in later life.

The **nephrotic syndrome**, in which there are continuing, and excessive, amounts of protein excreted in the urine, together with marked swelling of various parts of the body can also – but rarely – result from an attack of Henoch–Schonlein purpura.

THE FUTURE

Henoch–Schonlein purpura is rarely fatal. But if renal involvement has been severe, high blood pressure may be a problem in later life.

Impetigo

INCIDENCE

Impetigo is a well-known skin disease world-wide. Latterly – in the past decade – there has been an increase in the type of impetigo caused by a specific type of bacterium, with a decrease in impetigo cause by other bacteria.

Children are especially prone to this skin infection.

CAUSATION

Impetigo can be caused by either staphylococcal or streptococcal bacteria. As mentioned above, there has been a world-wide increase lately in impetigo caused by staphylococcal bacteria. Streptococcal impetigo is rarely seen nowadays. This has a bearing on the type of treatment necessary to cure the infection.

Impetigo often arises following other skin diseases such as eczema, scabies or even a minor insect bite. Scratching induced by these other skin conditions allows the bacteria to enter the abrased surface of the skin.

CHARACTERISTICS

Impetigo is an infection of the skin. Initially a small, blistery spot appears. The area around the mouth and nose is most frequently affected, although theoretically any part of the body can be affected. The skin in these former areas is more liable to infection because of the general soreness and irritation, with subsequent rubbing, caused by the common cold. The initial sore area increases with sometimes alarming rapidity, both in size and in the number of lesions. Within a few hours, the surface of the skin breaks down, leaving a raw, moist surface which quickly becomes crusted over. In a particular sub-type of impetigo, much serum is exuded from the broken-down rash. This forms a thick, yellow crust over an underlying reddened, sore area.

Impetigo is a highly **contagious** condition. In spite of the alarming sight of the rash of impetigo, this infection is not painful or itchy, and there is rarely any associated generalized systemic upset.

As the rash clears following treatment, superficial skin cells can sometimes be shed, leaving a raw area for a short time. This is known as the 'scalded skin syndrome' or 'Lyell's' disease. The rash of impetigo fortunately leaves no permanent scarring.

INVESTIGATIONS

Ideally a swab should be taken from the weeping lesion of impetigo and sent to the laboratory so that the invading organism can be identified. Using this information, the most suitable antibiotic can then be prescribed. This is especially important if a number of children – in a class, for example – are involved, or if the treatment given is not proving to be successful.

MANAGEMENT

As impetigo is caused by bacteria, **antibiotics** will soon clear the unpleasant rash. Whilst sensitivities to the particular organism are being awaited (or if it has not been possible to take a swab), erythromycin, given by mouth, is one of the most useful antibiotics.

In early stages, or where only a small area of skin is involved, an **antibiotic cream** may be sufficient to produce a cure.

School, and contact with other children, should be avoided until the lesions have completely cleared. Due to its highly infectious nature, impetigo can spread like wildfire through a class of schoolchildren or in a nursery. This is particularly so amongst the younger age groups due, in part, to their incomplete knowledge of hygiene at this age!

COMPLICATIONS

On the rare occasions that group A streptococcal bacteria are the cause of the impetigo, watch should be kept, for around 2 months after the infection, for possible kidney involvement. Signs of this will be:

- blood in the urine;
- swelling of tissues, particularly around the face;
- a decrease in the amount of urine passed.

This is a serious condition, and one which must receive urgent treatment. It must be stressed, however, that it is extremely rare – especially as impetigo due to streptococcal bacteria is unusual these days.

Impetigo may complicate a **pre-existing eczema**.

THE FUTURE

There are no long-term after-effects with an uncomplicated attack of impetigo. The condition can recur, as immunity to the bacteria is not gained from the one attack.

Lice

Alternative name

'Nits'

– this is not a true alternative name, as the 'nits' are the eggs of
the louse, but in common parlance – in Britain at least – many
people refer to lice by this colloquial name.

INCIDENCE

There are three types of known lice – the head louse, the body louse and
the 'crab' or pubic louse. The first two are similar but merely affect different
parts of the body – as evidenced by the name. The 'crab' or pubic louse is
a different, quite distinct species.

Lice occur world-wide, and are especially prominent in areas with low
standards of hygiene. The head louse is the one most commonly seen in Britain
and will be the type described.

The incidence of the head louse varies enormously from place to place
and from time to time with no obvious explanation for these facts. During
an 'epidemic' of infestation with the head louse, as many as 60% of children
in schools can be affected at any one time. A survey carried out in 1977
estimated that around 200 000 children in England were infected with head
lice – a sizeable problem.

Infestation is commonest in the 3–13-year age group, the incidence peak-
ing amongst the 6–9 year olds. Girls seem to be more commonly affected
than boys. Strangely enough, hair length seems to have little bearing on whether
lice are present or not. Both clean and dirty heads can be infested.

CAUSATION

Infestation is with the head louse. Although the head is most frequently, and
most heavily, infested, other hairy parts of the body can also be involved.

The insects live close to the roots of the hair, and feed on blood which they suck from the underlying skin. The female lays around six to eight eggs ('nits') every 24 hours. These nits are stuck firmly to the shafts of hair close to the scalp initially. (Obviously, as the hair grows, so the nits will be found lower down the shaft away from the head.) These hatch within about 10 days, and so the cycle is repeated, unless treatment to eradicate the lice – and the eggs – is given.

The female louse lives for about a month. So in this time around 240 eggs can be laid!

CHARACTERISTICS

There may be **no symptoms** at all in a child with a minimal number of head lice. The first clue to an infestation may be parents or school teachers seeing the characteristic white nits on the hair shafts.

Under conditions where there is a heavy infestation the child's head may **itch**. This irritation is probably due to an allergic reaction to the presence of the louse and not due to the movement of the insect. Children who are continually scratching their heads should be examined closely for the presence of lice. There are few other conditions in which there is such obvious irritation of the scalp alone. The most common places for the lice to congregate are behind the ears and on the back of the head.

The itching of the scalp can cause the child to be a **restless sleeper**, due to the constant low-grade irritation.

Excessive scratching of the scalp can cause an **infection** of the skin, giving rise to impetigo. This can lead to a mild **fever** and, in severe cases, enlargement of the **glands in the neck**. So any child with a mild fever and tender, swollen neck glands, but with no sore throat or other 'coldy' symptoms, should have the head examined for head lice. If impetigo has occurred due to excessive scratching, antibiotic treatment will be required.

Transmission of the head louse is by head-to-head contact. This, of course, is a very common event amongst small children, who frequently have their heads close together during play or during school activities. It is also thought that the lice can be passed on by the sharing of hair brushes and combs or by merely trying on the hats or other headgear of an infested playmate. Obviously, situations where there is overcrowding of children make for excellent conditions for the head louse to infect a number of children.

MANAGEMENT

On discovery of an infestation in one child, the whole class – including the teaching staff – should have their heads examined for lice. In Britain, the school health service usually undertakes this task when contacted by parents or teachers. (A decade or so ago, regular head inspections were all part of the routine health care in schools. This has now been suspended due to the professional time consumed for little apparent result. Control has been found to be better achieved by call-out when necessary.)

There are a number of preparations (**lotions** and **shampoos**) which effectively kill the head louse. The type used has to be changed in any one area at fairly frequent intervals due to the rapidity with which the louse becomes resistant to any one preparation. Good liaison between health authorities is necessary to preserve the efficacy of the preparations used.

The lotion or shampoo is applied to the child's head in the evening, allowed to dry naturally, and combed out the following morning. (The lotion is probably preferable to the shampoo.) This one treatment should effectively kill all the lice. But the nits can remain stuck to the shafts of the hair and may need combing out using a fine-toothed **nit comb**. The preparations used today are lethal to the nits as well as to the adult lice – so the combing is merely a cosmetic exercise.

There is no need to exclude the child from **school** once the treatment has been given. Every **family member**, including grandparents, should have the lotion applied to their hair once one child in the family is found to be infested – even if no lice or nits are found on other children or parents. This will ensure that no minute, lurking louse will survive. (Care must be taken that the lotion does not splash into the child's eyes, as it will cause severe irritation. Also, of course, care must be taken with the storage of the lotion – accidental ingestion by a toddler will need emergency treatment.)

PREVENTION

- Rapid and adequate **treatment** of the whole family once an infested member is found is the best way of prevention once an initial child is infected.
- Advising children not to borrow each other's **hats, combs etc.**
- Advice to parents on adequate and frequent brushing, combing and washing of children's hair.

Much emotion and upset can be caused by infestation with head lice in a school. But it must be remembered that once the lice are present in a class, they can just as easily jump onto a beautifully clean head as on to a less desirable one!

Limp

INCIDENCE

A limp can be a symptom of a number of conditions. So the incidence can only be recorded in connection with each specific condition. It is, however, vital that any child who limps for any significant period of time should be fully investigated.

CAUSATION

The causes of a limp in children can range from the trivial, such as a blister or a verruca somewhere on the foot, to the serious, such as a septic arthritis or a tumour. Signs and symptoms, with subsequent investigations and treatment, will be related to the causative factor.

CONDITIONS IN THE FEET

Conditions such as verrucae, blisters or a minor fracture following injury can cause a child to limp.

Blisters will need cleaning gently, but with no attempt to burst the blister if the skin is still intact. A simple Elastoplast dressing with removal of the offending footwear is all the treatment that is necessary. (If the covering skin is removed from a blister – either accidentally or on purpose – so exposing raw tissue, cellulitis can result. This inflammation of the connective tissues around the wound can spread alarmingly and affect the whole leg. Appropriate and rapid antibiotic treatment is necessary under these conditions.)

Verrucae are a particularly common finding in the 11–16-year age group, and can cause sufficient pain as to result in a limp at times. (This condition is dealt with under 'Warts'.)

Fractures of the small bones of the foot can occur, sometimes after a seemingly minor injury. If the child describes either a crushing or a twisting injury, and is still in pain a day or two after the event, medical advice should be sought. An X-ray will confirm, or exclude, this cause for a limp.

Foreign bodies in the foot are a common hazard of childhood, especially following barefoot physical exercise. Children will readily be able to point to the site of the implanted object. Removal will give relief and a return to a normal gait.

One of the **osteochondrites** (see under 'Perthes' disease') can affect the foot, causing a child to limp. **Sever's disease** is an osteochondritis of the heel, whilst **Kohler's disease** is a simlar problem affecting one of the tiny bones of the foot. The typical picture of osteochondritis can be seen on X-ray. Immobilization in plaster for 6–8 weeks may be necessary, although many milder cases will settle with a reduction in activity.

Juvenile chronic arthritis can first be manifest in the ankles. The child will complain of pain, and can limp in an endeavour to relieve this. This can be one of the first signs of the poly- or the pauciarticular types of juvenile arthritis. (See under 'Arthritis'.)

CONDITIONS IN THE HIP

Perthes' disease is a further example of one of the osteochondrites, this time affecting the hip. A limp can be the only sign of this condition for some time.

A **slipped femoral epiphysis** can be a further cause of a limp in an older child – usually in the early adolescent years. In this condition the growing head of the femur gradually slips until it is in a non-aligned position in relation to the pelvic bone. Occasionally the condition can occur suddenly as a result of a twisting injury. Under these circumstances the pain is acute and the boy or girl will be unable to move the affected leg. Boys are slightly more often affected than girls. Overweight children are thought to be more at risk from a slipped femoral epiphysis. As well as a limp, the young person is most likely to complain of pain in the knee – although the problem is in the hip. (Diseases of the hip often manifest themselves with pain referred to the knee joint. So any investigation of knee pain should include close examination of the hips.) On examination, there is swelling and limitation of the affected hip.

X-ray examination will confirm the diagnosis. Operative procedures are necessary to realign the head of the femur in the pelvis.

'**Irritable hip**' (transient synovitis) is a relatively common condition arising out of the blue with no known specific causative factor. The child will limp, and the muscles around the hip joint will be found to be in spasm. There may be an associated mild fever. Blood tests may also show a raised ESR (erythrocyte sedimentation rate). This condition usually settles adequately and quickly with a short period of bed rest.

MISCELLANEOUS CONDITIONS

One of the most potentially disabling causes of a long-term limp is an undiagnosed (in babyhood) **congenital dislocation of the hip**. Fortunately this is a rare occurrence in Britain today, with the routine examination of the hips of all babies at birth and at subsequent routine checks. But the possibility of this condition must always be remembered, particularly if the child has been born in a part of the world where such checks are not routinely performed.

Certain other – rare – conditions in which there is an **inequality in the leg length** can cause a limp. These include a congenitally shortened bone in a leg, or a scoliosis (a sideways twist in the spine due to a variety of causes). A previous attack of poliomyelitis can cause a shortening of one leg – again a rare cause these days in the developed countries, but still to be remembered in a child who has lived in a country where poliomyelitis is still endemic.

The possibility of a **tumour** – benign or malignant – in one of the leg bones must also be considered. Pain and swelling over the site are the most usual manifestations, but a limp can also be one of the first signs in a younger child. Further investigations, followed by appropriate treatment, must be instigated rapidly if a tumour is suspected.

Finally, the possibilty of **non-accidental injury** must always be considered in a child with a limp. Careful examination of the whole of the child's body must be undertaken, with follow-up X-rays if necessary, to exclude injuries for which there is no rational explanation.

Most limps in children are due to trivial and obvious causes. But important and treatable diseases can be missed if a long-term limp is ignored.

Measles

Alternative name

Rubeola.

INCIDENCE

Notification of this disease began in 1940, and the number of cases reported was high in the decades up to the mid-1960s. It was at this time that immunization against measles was introduced. As many as 800 000 children every year suffered from this infection before the advent of immunization. At this time the incidence of the disease showed a marked biannual variation, every other year being a 'bad' measles year.

Since the introduction of the measles vaccine in the mid-1960s the incidence of the infection has fallen dramatically, the 1970s and 1980s averaging around 100 000 notifications or less every year.

In 1988 the MMR (measles, mumps and rubella) vaccine was started and given routinely to all babies between the first and second years of life. Since this time, the notification of cases of measles has dropped to the low 100's every year.

Measles occurs most frequently in the 5–10-year age group, although in crowded urban conditions younger children are seen to contract the infection. Measles is extremely rare under the age of 6 months. Antibodies from the mother protect the baby from the infection during these critical early months of life.

In developing countries, who have not experienced the benefit of the measles vaccine and in whose children malnutrition is an every-present problem, measles is a potent killer disease. As many as 25% of children die from this infection.

Although measles, like many of the other so-called 'childhood' infections, is comparatively mild today, complications can – and do – still occur. There are, regretfully, still a few deaths in the UK every year attributable to measles. Children who have other serious conditions, such as leukaemia, are especially at risk.

HISTORY

In some parts of rural Africa today, babies are not given a name until the expected measles epidemic has passed. The death rate is so high amongst young children that parents feel that they cannot risk positively identifying their child until he or she has successfully survived the measles epidemic.

CAUSATION

Measles is caused by a virus, and is a highly infectious condition. Transmission is by droplet infection from the respiratory tract. The infection is usually passed on before the typical rash appears, and hence before a definite diagnosis of measles is made.

The incubation period is between 8 and 14 days.

CHARACTERISTICS

Measles begins in much the same way as does any common cold, namely:

1. a **runny nose**, associated with catarrhal symptoms;
2. sore, inflamed **eyes** with marked photophobia (a dislike of light);
3. a harsh, dry **cough**;
4. a **fever** of varying degree;
5. general **malaise**;
6. **convulsions**, which sometimes occur due to the high fever.

These are very generalized symptoms which can initially be thought to be due to a number of causes, e.g. the curren tupper respiratory tract infection that is 'going the rounds'. But within 2 or 3 days, a very specific sign of measles can be noted in the child's mouth. Small white spots, which have been likened to grains of salt, appear on the insides of the cheeks opposite the back teeth. These are known as **Koplik spots** and only occur with an infection with the measles virus.

On the third or fourth day of the illness the diagnosis becomes obvious, with the appearance of the typical **rash**. This rash starts behind the ears and along the hair-line. It spreads rapidly to involve the whole body and limbs, the face and upper chest being usually most affected. The dusky red spots coalesce, giving rise to a blotchy appearance.

The rash begins to fade after 3 or 4 days, often with some shedding of the surface skin. (This is rather like the desquamation seen in scarlet fever. In measles, however, the hands and feet are not involved in this process.)

With the appearance of the rash, a high **fever** can recur. This will improve as the rash fades. In uncomplicated cases of measles, improvement is rapid following the disappearance of the rash, and within a week, in mild cases, the child will be returned to full health. Occasionally the dry cough will persist for a week or two.

INVESTIGATIONS

These are rarely, if ever, needed to make a diagnosis of measles, as the signs and symptoms are so definite once the rash has appeared. The virus can be isolated and grown from the secretions of the nose and throat as well as from the urine of a sufferer.

COMPLICATIONS

It is the complications that can occur with measles that make this infection so potentially dangerous. For descriptive purposes, it is convenient to look at these in relationship to the body system involved.

Respiratory tract

There is always an associated respiratory involvement with an attack of measles. The trachea (windpipe), larynx and bronchi are all involved in this viral infection, as is evidenced in the sore throat and dry cough. Secondary infection with bacteria is an ever-present threat when these tissues are damaged by the measles virus. Bronchitis is an almost inevitable accompaniment to measles, and pneumonia is a common complication.

Symptoms of further involvement of the respiratory tract will include:

- a return of **fever**;
- a worsening of the **cough**.

Further medical advice should always be sought if these symptoms should occur in a child who is getting over an attack of measles. Antibiotics, and maybe hospital admission, will be necessary under these circumstances.

Central nervous system

Convulsions can occur during the early stages of the infection. Medical advice should always be sought for a child who has had a convulsion.

Encephalitis (inflammation of the brain) is the most serious complication of measles. The time at which signs and symptoms appear can vary, but most usually they occur around 7–10 days after the beginning of the illness. The child will become **drowsy**, suffer from **convulsions** and have a return of the

fever. Specific neurological signs may also occur such as weakening or paralysis of a limb. This serious state of affairs can either:

- show a steady slow improvement with no permanent after-effects;
- show a slow recovery, but leave the child with permanent neurological and/or intellectual damage;
- show a steady deterioration resulting in a fatal outcome.

A rare form of encephalitis can occur some 5–10 years after an attack of measles. This is known as 'sub-acute sclerosing panencephalitis, and is an extremely serious condition. The child at first shows some falling-off of intellectual abilities, together with some instability of posture and difficulty in movement. This vicious condition progresses inexorably into paralysis and dementia and finally coma and death. This condition is thought to be due to a reactivation, by some unknown stimulus, of the measles virus which has remained latent in the brain.

Eyes

The **conjunctiva** of the eye is involved to some degree in every case of measles, as is evidenced by the photophobia complained of by most children with measles.

As with the respiratory tract, secondary bacterial infection can occur, resulting in irritation of the cornea.

Ears

Otitis media used to be an almost invariable accompaniment to measles. **Earache** and high **fever** with possible rupture of the eardrum and/or mastoiditis added to the miseries of the child with measles. Fortunately, today, with the seemingly lower virulence of the measles virus as well as prompt antibiotic treatment, this is an unusual complication.

Gastrointestinal tract

The whole of the gut seems to be involved in the measles infection, ranging from soreness in the mouth to indigestion and abdominal pain. As well as direct involvement of the gut in the generalized infection, lymph glands in the abdomen are also enlarged by the infective process – yet one further uncomfortable and unpleasant aspect of this viral disease!

MANAGEMENT

This will obviously be different for the child with complications and for the child suffering from an uncomplicated attack of measles.

Uncomplicated measles

Adequate **rest** is needed, in bed during the initial stages of the infection if symptoms are at all severe. When the child's temperature has settled and energy is returning, quiet play in a warm room is satisfactory.

An adequate **fluid** intake is necessary to ensure that the child does not become dehydrated. High fever causes fluid loss through perspiration, and also unwillingness to eat and drink causes dehydration. Food should not be forced on the child, but plenty of drinks – of any kind – should be encouraged.

Paracetamol, in any form in appropriate dosage, will help to lower temperature as well as relieving headache and sore throat.

Whilst a **darkened room** will not in any way improve the sore eyes so commonly associated with measles, the child will probably feel more comfortable in subdued light. Soothing eye-drops can also be prescribed.

Antibiotics have no part to play in an uncomplicated attack of measles. (These drugs are not active against viral infections.) But if there is any suggestion of secondary bacterial infection anywhere in the body, antibiotics should be prescribed.

Complicated attack of measles

Antibiotics, usually penicillin, will be needed if respiratory or ear involvement occurs.

Neurological involvement will usually necessitate admission to hospital for nursing, monitoring and an adequate nutrition programme.

Long-term management of the results of complications of measles will depend on how much permanent damage has been done.

Neurological and/or **intellectual** problems will need regular review for many months, as improvement can be maintained for some time after the initial infection has subsided. Intellectual abilities will also need regular assessment and review, with special schooling arranged if necessary.

Hearing should be checked a month or so after full recovery if the ears have been involved to any degree. Children can be left with varying degrees of deafness after measles, and it is important that this is recognized and appropriate help given.

Measles is an unpleasant disease with potent serious complications, and should never be taken lightly. Fortunately, with the advent of immunization against the disease the incidence has reduced dramatically. Nevertheless, measles does still occur and will continue to do so until at least 90% of children have benefited from the vaccine.

Even mild cases can leave a child debilitated. It is wise to avoid too many active pursuits for a week or two after recovery, and to ensure that the convalescent child receives adequate rest and nutrition.

PREVENTION

Prevention is by immunization. This is done routinely in the UK today between 1 and 2 years of age with the MMR (measles, mumps and rubella) vaccine. This vaccine should be given even if the child has been thought to have had an attack of naturally occurring measles previously. Age is no bar to receiving this vaccine if it has been missed at the usual time.

Contraindications to receiving the vaccine are the usual ones of:

- an acute feverish illness at the time when the immunization is due – the vaccine should be given when the child has recovered;
- any form of malignant disease or treatment with immunosuppressant drugs for any reason.

Allergy to eggs at one time caused much alarm amongst mothers, and many children were denied the benefits of the vaccine merely because they disliked eggs. The only reason for not giving the vaccine in this context is if the child has a **severe** reaction when eating eggs – such as swelling of the mouth and throat or difficulty in breathing.

THE FUTURE

At attack of measles confers immunity for life. Apart from the rare possibility of sub-acute sclerosing panencephalitis, or neurological or hearing damage from one of the complications, there are no other adverse effects in later life from an attack of measles.

When immunization levels of children have reached the advised target, measles should be an infection of the past as is, for example, poliomyelitis today. But meanwhile children can still suffer from measles. It must also be remembered that measles is still a common, and much-feared, disease in developing countries, and, with today's ease of travel, unimmunized people are at risk of acquiring the infection.

Meningitis

INCIDENCE

Meningitis is caused by a wide variety of viruses and bacteria. The viruses that can cause meningitis are numerous and so the exact incidence of cases of viral meningitis is difficult to determine.

Bacterial meningitis also has a large number of responsible bacteria (see below). Figures for meningococcal meningitis are well documented and the illness due to this cause can be seen to occur in peaks. For example, in the early 1970s over 1000 cases were notified. In the early 1980s these figures fell to around 400, but in the late 1980s notifications were again as high as 1300 cases.

Meningitis due to bacteria is essentially an infection of childhood, and over 80% of all notified cases are in children under the age of 15 years. A high majority of these occur in children under the age of 5 years.

CAUSATION

The **viruses** capable of causing meningitis are multiple. They range from such viruses as those causing measles and mumps through the common ECHO and Coxsackie viruses to other specific viruses such as herpes simplex and Epstein–Barr viruses – a formidable list!

The **bacteria** capable of causing meningitis are less numerous, but there is still a not inconsiderable number. In the early days of life, meningitis is more often due to infection with certain types of **streptococcal** bacteria, *E. coli* and the *Haemophilus influenzae* B bacteria. *Haemophilus influenzae* B is the commonest cause of meningitis in the 1–4-year age group.

CHARACTERISTICS

Whatever the infecting agent causing the illness, the characteristics (with a few exceptions) seen are similar.

Headache and/or **pain at the back of the neck** are two of the most frequent early features. Associated with the pain at the back of the neck is a reluctance to bend the head forward. For example, if children are asked to 'kiss their knees' they are unable to do so without an exacerbation of the pain in the back of the neck.

Nausea and vomiting – unassociated with abdominal pain – are also a common feature. The vomiting can be projectile in character.

Fever of varying degree is the usual accompaniment to these symptoms.

Photophobia (a dislike of light) can be marked, with the child turning away from the window and burying his or her face in the pillow.

Drowsiness and **irritability** on being disturbed can occur within a few hours. **Convulsions** can also occur.

With a specific type of meningitis – meningococcal meningitis – there is an associated **rash**. This is very specific, and consists of numerous small bruiselike spots all over the body. This is a sign of a serious infection which can be rapidly fatal – within hours – unless treatment is given.

In younger children, under 2 years, these characteristic signs are not so well marked. **Fever, vomiting** and **pallor** together with a **high-pitched cry** and **refusal of feeds** can be all that is noticed initially. **Drowsiness** and/or **convulsions** are later serious signs in these younger children.

INVESTIGATIONS

A **lumbar puncture** to obtain cerebrospinal fluid must be performed, in hospital, before treatment is started. (There is one major exception to this. If meningococcal meningitis is suspected – the specific rash being a strong diagnostic feature – immediate treatment with intramuscular penicillin must be given before removal to hospital.) The cerebrospinal fluid thus obtained is seen to be cloudy in cases of meningitis. Laboratory examination will be able to determine the infecting agent.

Blood tests to determine the infecting agent are also useful.

MANAGEMENT

The child with meningitis can be seriously ill, and will often need to be admitted to hospital, where the following treatments are given.

● **Antibiotic** treatment is begun immediately after the cerebrospinal fluid has been obtained by lumbar puncture. (The reason why treatment is not started before this investigation is done – except, of course, in the case of suspected meningococcal meningitis – is that the treatment can confuse the laboratory diagnosis of which infecting agent is present.) Penicillin and/or chloramphenicol are the most usual antibiotics used, and it is usual to continue to give these drugs for at least 10 days.

- **Fluids**, intravenously initially, can be necessary. The young child can become rapidly dehydrated if vomiting and fever are severe. Refusal to eat or drink also results in lack of fluid in the body.

Regular **monitoring** of the child's temperature, pulse, respiration and level of consciousness is also an important necessity. If there is any deterioration shown by these regular readings, immediate help can be given.

If convulsions have occurred, or if the child is extremely restless, **anticonvulsant** drugs may be necessary for a short while.

Parents will need **emotional support** and maybe also **physical help** (with other children or with travelling to hospital, for example) during their child's serious illness.

With an uncomplicated attack of meningitis, recovery is complete with no permanent after-effects. Following discharge from hospital, it is wise to allow the child a week or two of convalescence before returning to the rough and tumble of the school day. Extra rest and a nutritious diet will help to restore general health.

COMPLICATIONS

Serious long-term complications can occur following a severe attack of meningitis. Probably the most common complication is a **sensorineural deafness**. From studies on the complications of meningitis, around 10% of children are found to have some degree of deafness following the disease. This would appear to depend very much on the organism causing the infection. Infection with streptococcal bacteria was shown in one study to affect hearing in 30% of the children suffering from this type of meningitis.

All children should have their hearing tested a month or two after recovery from meningitis. Hearing aids and/or special schooling may be needed with the more severe cases. It is important that good liaison is maintained between health and education authorities involved with these children.

Epilepsy can be a late complication of meningitis. There does not appear to be any correlation between later epilepsy and the type of infecting organism. Children who have had convulsions during the intitial stages of their illness are most likely to develop later epilepsy. It is thought that this complication affects around 5% of children following meningitis. Anticonvulsant drugs will be necessary to control seizures.

Mental retardation can regretfully be a sequel to meningitis. The child's abilities (at school if a school-age child) will be seen to have fallen off since the illness. In pre-school children, skills previously learned may be lost, and only regained slowly. Regular developmental checks are necessary for the pre-school child to determine the extent of the damage. These should be repeated regularly over succeeding months, as recovery can continue for some time after the acute stage of the illness is over. Again, special educational facilities may be required, with close liaison between health and education authorities.

Cerebral palsy, in which there are problems with control of the muscles of the body, can also occur after an attack of meningitis. Limbs can either become stiff and rigid with much difficulty in walking, or become floppy and weak. Here again, regular assessment by a paediatrician, skilled in handicapping motor conditions, is vital. Physiotherapy is also important to enable the child to make the most of residual abilities. Speech problems may be also part of the picture, and help from a speech therapist is invaluable under these cicumstances.

Mental handicap and/or cerebral palsy are thought to affect 3–8% of children following an attack of meningitis.

PREVENTION

One form of meningitis is now preventable by **immunization**. This is the meningitis due to the *Haemophilus influenzae* B bacterium – the most common type of meningitis seen in children between the ages of 1 and 4 years.

Immunization with this vaccine is part of the routine babyhood immunization schedule in the UK. Three injections of the vaccine, at monthly intervals, are given at the same time as the triple vaccine (against diphtheria, tetanus and whooping cough) at 2, 3 and 4 months of age. This affords protection for the child over the years when infection with this type of organism is at its height. Work is progressing on combining this vaccine with the triple vaccine. There are no contraindications to a baby receiving this vaccine, apart from the usual ones of an acute illness (when the immunization should be postponed) or if there has been a severe reaction to a previous dose of vaccine. These reactions are virtually unknown. No serious reaction has been reported after the giving of over 20 million doses of this vaccine. Minor reactions, such as redness and swelling around the injection site for a few hours, do occur, but resolve rapidly.

There are no vaccines, or other preventable methods, against meningitis due to other infective organisms.

Outbreaks of meningococcal meningitis in nurseries or schools will need public health advice as to the advisability of giving penicillin, or vaccine, to children in close contact with the sufferer from this form of meningitis.

THE FUTURE

Following at attack of meningitis in childhood, there are no deleterious after-effects unless complications – as discussed above – have occurred. These, of course, can be severe, needing long-term specialized help.

SELF-HELP GROUP

National Meningitis Trust
Fern House
Bath Road
Stroud
Gloucester GL5 3TJ
(Tel. 0453 751738)

Migraine

INCIDENCE

Migraine is rare under the age of 2 years. The incidence of this unpleasant condition increases with age, until by school age around 50 children in every 1000 are thought to have suffered from an attack of migraine at one time or another.

Before puberty the number of boys suffering from migraine is about twice the number of girls. At puberty, however, the number of male sufferers decreases and that of females increases until the adult incidence of excess attacks in women is reached. This indicates that this alteration in incidence must have some relationship to hormonal changes occuring around the time of puberty.

HISTORY

Socrates gave accounts of classical migraine around 25 centuries ago, so migraine is certainly not a new environmental disease!

Lewis Carroll of *Alice in Wonderland* fame was known to have suffered from severe attacks of migraine. Hallucinations of becoming smaller and smaller – so graphically described in his works – are typical of a certain specific late effect of migraine.

CAUSATION

Migraine is thought to be due to alterations in the reactions of the blood vessels supplying the brain. There is a phase when these vessels constrict and become smaller and so reduce the blood supply to a particular part of the brain. A subsequent phase occurs when the vessels dilate and the blood supply is increased. Different blood vessels can be affected at different times. This probably accounts for the wide variety of symptoms seen in this condition.

These effects on the blood vessels are due in turn to a wide variety of stimuli. These range from genetic susceptibility through reaction to certain foods and exercise to possible hormonal imbalance and reaction to viral infections.

Genetic predisposition: it has been found that 90% of children suffering from migraine have one or more members of the immediate family who also suffer from this condition.

Foods that are most often implicated in the onset of an attack of migraine are cheese and chocolate, with oranges a close third. The two former foods contain a substance, tyramine, which is a powerful dilator of blood vessels.

Monosodium glutamate has also been blamed, and may be the cause of the attacks of migraine from which some people suffer following the eating of a Chinese meal. This substance, a flavour enhancer, is an ingredient in many – delicious – Chinese dishes.

Milk products, eggs and gluten-containing foods (gluten being the product found in wheat and wheat products) have at times also been considered to precipitate attacks of migraine. These foods may, of course, also precipitate other conditions (such as coeliac disease, which results from an allergy to gluten) and the migraine may be but one symptom of a generalized food intolerance.

Exercise, particularly if associated with competitive sports, may precipitate migraine in some children. It can be difficult to decide whether it is the exercise itself or the worry of the competition that causes the problem! (Again, under these circumstances, true migraine can easily be confused with the so-called 'tension' headaches, although the latter are rare before adolescence.)

Sex hormones, androgens and oestrogens, are probably responsible for the change in incidence of migraine seen at puberty. The extra androgens secreted by boys around the time of puberty appear to reduce the tendency to migraine, whilst oestrogens in higher levels in girls after puberty appear to increase the tendency. Changes in oestrogen levels at various times in the menstrual cycle also influence the timing of attacks in some girls.

It is possible that a **viral infection** can precipitate an attack of migraine in a susceptible individual. This may be difficult to differentiate from the headache due to the infection itself in children. (With age and experience, the person suffering from migraine will be only too well aware of the difference)

Considering the number of possible causes, it is no wonder that migraine is so difficult to control!

CHARACTERISTICS

Migraine, for descriptive purposes, can be divided into a number of subsections – each due to changes in the blood vessels, but with slightly differing symptoms.

Classical migraine has a very definite 'aura' followed by a one-sided headache. This aura usually takes the form of visual manifestations, but specific smells have also been described. The visual aura can consist, for example, of blurring of the vision or flashes of light compounded by a zig-zag pattern. Also, some people experience an absence of part of their visual field, leaving words and sentences chopped in half. These visual effects are found in around 30% of children with migraine, and can be very worrying to the child when they are first experienced. The headache usually follows on after the visual manifestations, or it can arise at the same time.

Common migraine is less likely to be associated with an aura. The headache is also not so likely to be felt on one side of the head, but more as a generalized headache. Nausea and/or vomiting can accompany this type of migraine as well as general feelings of malaise.

Complicated migraine is said to occur when attacks of giddiness and/or periodic attacks of vomiting ('cyclical vomiting' or 'abdominal migraine') occur. The headache under these circumstances is not the most prominent feature. Children with this type of cyclical vomiting – which can also be accompanied by abdominal pain – frequently go on to develop the more usual forms of migraine in later life.

It can be difficult to differentiate the attacks of giddiness from epilepsy, as the child can be so dizzy as to fall to the ground during an attack.

Children with any form of migraine also appear to suffer from **travel sickness** more frequently than do other children, the figures being quoted as about 40%.

INVESTIGATIONS

It is important that, before settling on a diagnosis of migraine, other physical causes for the headache are excluded. Other serious conditions which could be the cause of the headache in children are brain tumours, continued bleeding into the brain following even a mild head injury, a raised blood pressure or a previously undiagnosed hydrocephalus (an excess of fluid found in specialized cavities of the brain).

As a brief guide, any child with a combination of

- a headache which is worse on waking from sleep;
- a headache which wakes him from sleep;
- a headache which is worse on coughing;
- persistent visual problems, such as seeing coloured lights or zig-zag lines for several days;
- a behavioural change for no obvious reason;
- neurological symptoms such as weakness, for example, of any part of the body;
- no family history of migraine

should be further investigated to find the reason for the headaches. (Other less serious causes such as sinusitis should also be excluded before a diagnosis of migraine is arrived at.) Investigations under these circumstances include:

- checking on the **blood pressure** after a careful history of the type and timing of the headaches has been taken;
- an **electroencephalogram**, especially if the child becomes drowsy or confused in association with the headaches;
- a **CT scan** if symptoms suggest that the headaches may be due to a serious and treatable cause.

If none of the pointers suggests a cause other than migraine, a few simple investigations will help to identify 'triggering' factors:

- relationship to stressful events – even such enjoyable ones as birthday parties or theatre visits as well as the more obvious ones of competitive sports or exams of any kind, for example;
- discussion with schoolteachers regarding the child's progress in school – worries about difficulties in certain areas of schooling may be causing the child frustration which is showing itself by headaches.

MANAGEMENT

Many of the migraine attacks suffered by both children and adults can be aborted by **lying down** in a darkened, quiet room for an hour. This is most frequently successful if this action is taken before the attack is fully developed. Children who are used to attacks of migraine will known when an attack is imminent. Sympathetic parents and/or teachers (particularly those who suffer from migraine themselves) will encourage the child to lie down as soon as symptoms become obvious.

Analgesics, such as paracetamol compounds, will also shorten an attack if taken early enough, particularly if combined with a period of rest.

Anti-emetic drugs, such as prochlorperazine, are useful if nausea and vomiting are a problem. Again, if they are taken at the first warning signs of an attack the effect can be greater.

Children with 'cyclical vomiting' – a special type of complicated migraine – can benefit from regular treatment with one of the anti-emetic drugs. This can be especially helpful during a period of stress when attacks of vomiting and/or headache occur with monotonous regularity.

Drugs acting directly on the **blood vessels** are also available. Their use for children, however, is limited due to both the type of migraine commonly suffered by children and to the side-effects of these drugs. Only in intractable migraine, and then under strict medical supervision, are these drugs used.

Biofeedback techniques have been tried with some children with varying degrees of success. Here, measurement of the skin resistance and blood flow followed by techniques to alter these are used.

Elimination diets can also be tried for children in whom other methods have failed and there is thought to be a food component.

Common-sense handling of the attacks by all adults involved with the child is also of importance. Too much emphasis on the migraine will cause concern, and hence further attacks. The difficult balancing act between sympathetic understanding and encouragement is an art to be learned by all parents of children who suffer from migraine.

PREVENTION

Choosing to be born into a **family** who have no idea of what a migrainous headache is like is probably the best – but completely unattainable! – way to prevent migraine.

Avoidance of **foods** which are known to bring on an attack is also an obvious way of prevention.

Stressful situations can also to a certain extent be controlled as the child matures and becomes more in control of both environment and stressful situations.

Checking on the possibility of **learning difficulties**, with remedial teaching made available if this is positive, can do much to relieve the stress of repeated failure.

THE FUTURE

Migraine fortunately tends to decrease both in frequency and severity with age, but this may not occur until early middle age has been reached. The teenage years and the 20s and 30s can be trying, but experience will show how best to avoid or abort attacks.

Mumps

Alternative name

Epidemic parotitis.

INCIDENCE

Until 1988, mumps was not a notifiable disease in Britain, so accurate figures on the number of children contracting the disease are not available. Hospital records show, however, that about 1200 admissions to hospital each year in England and Wales were due to mumps or one of the complications of the infection.

Children of both sexes between the ages of 5 and 15 years are the usual sufferers from an attack of mumps. It is rare in children below the age of 5 years.

HISTORY

Mumps has been mentioned historically for many years. In fact, 'mump' is an old English word meaning 'mope' – a good description of someone with the uncomfortably swollen face that accompanies this infection.

CAUSATION

Mumps is an infectious disease of the salivary glands caused by a specific virus. The parotid salivary glands, situated on each side of the face below and in front of the ears, are the glands most commonly – and obviously – affected. The other salivary glands, beneath the chin and tongue, are also frequently affected.

The condition is spread by droplet infection from the breath of a sufferer. Children are infectious for several days before the obvious signs of mumps appear. The incubation period of the disease is 14–21 days. The infection can be passed on for several days after the swelling of the glands becomes apparent.

Immunity to the virus is life-long following an attack of mumps.

CHARACTERISTICS

As with many of the infectious 'childhood' fevers, mumps can begin with the very general symptoms of **headache**, **fever**, **loss of appetite** and a general feeling of ill-health – all very non-specific. But within 2–3 days, the diagnosis will become obvious when **pain** and **swelling** in the parotid glands (and maybe the other salivary glands as well) occur. Occasionally the swelling can be the first sign of the condition, the usual prodromal symptoms being absent. Either one or both of the parotid glands can be involved. The swellings may be small or very large and extremely painful and tender. Sometimes the swelling on one side of the face will disappear, only for the opposite parotid gland to become swollen. The types of symptoms that occur will make no difference to the immunity gained by an accurately diagnosed attack of mumps.

Eating or **drinking** can cause exquisite pain in the affected glands at the height of the infection. A **dry mouth** is also a common complaint with an attack of mumps. This is due to the reduction in the amounts of saliva secreted by the affected salivary glands.

INVESTIGATIONS

Identification of the virus in the laboratory from saliva swabs gives positive proof of infection with mumps virus. However, this is rarely done, as diagnosis can usually be made on clinical grounds.

MANAGEMENT

There is no specific treatment for an attack of mumps.

Analgesics are necessary to control the pain in cases where the parotid glands are swollen and tender. It is a good idea to give a painkiller about half-an-hour before a meal in order to reduce the pain caused by the attempted salivary secretion by the inflamed gland. These useful drugs – such as paracetamol – will also help to lower fever, and so make the young patient feel more comfortable.

A suitable **diet** is also helpful during the height of an attack of mumps. Fluids only at the height of the swelling may be necessary. After this, easily swallowed foods such as soups, jellies, ice-cream and liquidized foods are suggested.

Children will need to remain **off school** until the worst of the swelling of the parotid glands has subsided. Infectivity is high until 4–5 days after the appearance of the swellings. After this time, schooling can be resumed with no risk to children in contact with the sufferer, always provided, of course, that the child is feeling completely well again.

COMPLICATIONS

Mumps has a poor record where complications are concerned. Indeed this is an important factor in an otherwise mild infectious disease.

Meningitis can occur due to the mumps virus. Occasionally, signs and symptoms of meningitis can be the first clue that a child is suffering from infection with the mumps virus. At other times, the meningitis occurs along with the swelling in the parotid glands or, again, after the worst of the swelling has subsided – as long as 10 days later. So this complication can be very variable in its onset.

Signs of meningitis are **fever** (or a return of fever once the fever due to the original infection has subsided), **headache**, a **stiff neck** and, at times, a **sore throat**.

Hospital admission is usually necessary for a child with mumps meningitis. A lumbar puncture will confirm the diagnosis following laboratory examination of the cerebrospinal fluid thus obtained. As a side-effect, the lumbar puncture can bring rapid relief to headache.

Again, there is no specific treatment for mumps meningitis apart from good nursing care. (Antibiotics are of no value, as they are inactive against viral infections.)

Recovery is usually complete, but sadly occasional permanent brain damage can result from severe mumps meningitis.

Unilateral deafness can also be a residual handicap following mumps. Children who have had a severe attack of mumps in whom deafness is suspected by the parents, or any child who has suffered from meningitis due to this infection, should receive a hearing test a few weeks following recovery from the infection. It can be all too easy to miss this complication, particularly in the younger age groups.

Orchitis is a further possible complication to an attack of mumps, but is rare before puberty. Here, one or both testes become acutely painful, red and swollen. Treatment is again non-specific. Support of the inflamed testes with appropriate firm bandages can be helpful, as can ice-bags applied to the hot swollen organ. Frequent painkillers can also be necessary. Sterility is by no means the inevitable outcome of a mumps orchitis, as was once thought. Mothers of young boys should be firmly reassured on this point.

Pancreatitis, in which the pancreas becomes involved in the general infection, is a rare complication, but can be the cause of acute abdominal pain during an attack of mumps. There is usually no permanent damage to this organ, but, very occasionally, diabetes can subsequently occur.

PREVENTION

Immunization against mumps is now possible with the MMR (measles, mumps and rubella) vaccine. This immunization is now a routine procedure in Britain at the age of around 1–2 years. Only one injection is necessary to ensure immunity. There is a risk of other members of the family acquiring any of the three infections from a younger, recently immunized, member.

Immunization should be postponed if the child due to receive the injection has any acute illness. Also, children receiving immunotherapy for other serious illnesses should not be given this immunization. The only other contraindication to receiving the vaccine is a proven allergy to the antibiotic neomycin or a serious reaction after eating eggs. (Egg products are used in the making of the vaccine.) Mere dislike of eggs is no reason for omitting the vaccine! The immunization can be given to children of any age.

THE FUTURE

With the advent of immunization against mumps, this infection should eventually become an historical disease. In the USA, mumps vaccine has been given to children for over 20 years, and there has been a dramatic drop in the number of infections and the complications due to mumps reported. The most important factor must, of course, be the number of children suffering permanent consequences due to a severe complicated attack of mumps.

Otitis media

As with tonsillitis, for example, the true incidence of otitis media is not formally known. But any general practitioner will see a number of children every week with this condition. Boys and girls of all races are equally affected.

The incidence of this infection is higher in cool, temperate climates during the winter months, when upper respiratory infections are at their height. Throat infections and/or tonsillitis frequently precede, or coexist, with acute otitis media.

HISTORY

Until routine treatment of otitis media with antibiotics from around the 1950s onwards, mastoiditis (infection in the bony mastoid process) was a relatively common condition. The mastoid process is situated behind and below the ears. This bony process readily becomes infected following a severe, untreated otitis media. This infection was a serious side-effect of otitis media with meningitis as a further possible sequel. Operation on the mastoid process was necessary to remove and drain the infected bone. Older people still show the scars of this procedure along with the deafness that was often also the residual result.

CAUSATION

The infecting organisms in otitis media can be either bacteria or viruses. Probably around half of the infections are due to a viral cause, but secondary bacterial infection is common.

CHARACTERISTICS

Pain in the ear is the outstanding feature of acute otitis media. Even very young children accurately pinpoint the source of their pain as they clasp a hand over the affected ear, or rub their ear along a blanket or sheet. This pain can be one of the reasons for frequent waking in the night.

Fever, sometimes high, is also a frequent accompaniment of an acute ear infection. Associated **coughs** and **colds** are again common. This is due to the easy spread of the infection, up the Eustachian tube, into the middle ear.

On examination with an auroscope, the **eardrum** is seen to be reddened and covered with **dilated blood vessels** in early stages of the infection. Later the delicate tissue of the drum will appear unusually **dull** and **congested** and be bulging into the external auditory meatus. Ultimately, if no treatment has been available, the eardrum can **rupture** into the external auditory meatus. When this occurs, the pain will ease (due to the release of pressure) and a discharge of blood and pus will be seen flowing from the affected ear. Otitis media should never be allowed to reach this stage. Deafness can be a permanent late effect of rupture of the eardrum. The scar tissue which replaces the hole in the drum reduces the elasticity, and hence the adequate function, of this vital part of the hearing mechanism.

MANAGEMENT

Earache in children must always be regarded as an emergency, and medical help sought as soon as possible. Early treatment with **antibiotics** is essential if permanent damage to hearing is to be avoided. The pain from most attacks of otitis media usually clears up within 24 hours of starting treatment. But, in spite of this, it is important that the full course of prescribed antibiotic should be finished, in order that the infection is fully eradicated.

If the pain does not subside after a couple of days of treatment with a specific antibiotic, it will be necessary to change to a different one – and so, once again, medical advice should be sought.

Analgesics, such as paracetamol, should be given in the early painful stages of otitis media. This will also help to reduce fever.

A **hearing test** should ideally be performed 3 months or so after a severe attack of otitis media. This is to ensure that the infection has not left the child with the complication of **secretory otitis media** ('glue ear').

CAUSATION

The cause of secretory otitis media, as well as the possibility of this arising following an acute attack of otitis media, is unclear. It is thought that it is perhaps due to lack of proper drainage, via the Eustachian tube, of secretions. This tiny tube can easily become blocked by mucus, or by swelling of the surrounding tissues, and so cause a build-up of sticky fluid in the middle ear.

In turn, this fluid restricts the movement of the eardrum, so preventing sound waves from travelling clearly to the nerves of hearing.

CHARACTERISTICS

Secretory otitis media can be difficult to pinpoint. A child's hearing can be perfectly normal for several days, but for the next week or two can be very restricted due to a further build-up of fluid. The first signs of hearing loss can be lack of attention in school, or turning up the sound on the television to an unusually high level. Behavioural problems, too, can have their basis in a hearing loss. The unfortunate child cannot hear clearly what is being said in class, becomes frustrated and so 'switches off' altogether or reacts in a generally antisocial manner. In younger children with this problem, the proper development of speech can be hindered.

INVESTIGATIONS

If secretory otitis media is suspected, an ear, nose and throat surgeon should see the child, to examine the eardrum and to perform specialized hearing tests such as impedance audiometry.

MANAGEMENT

This can be difficult, but includes trying:

1. **anticongestant** nose drops;
2. **antihistamine drugs**.

Both these treatments have been prescribed over the years, but regretfully both can be less than satisfactory.

Myringotomy involves the eardrum being pierced, under a general anaesthetic, and the sticky fluid being withdrawn. Following this, a tiny ventilation tube, or 'grommet', is placed in the eardrum to allow air into the cavity of the middle ear and so prevent the repeated build-up of fluid.

'Grommets' rarely, if ever, need to be removed from their position in the eardrum. They fall out spontaneously, usually within a year to 18 months of their insertion. (They are so tiny that parents are usually quite unaware that they have been extruded. It is not until the ears are again examined with an auroscope that the grommets are found to be missing.)

There has been much controversy over the years regarding the vexed question of whether or not children with grommets in their ears should be allowed to swim. It is unlikely that any harm will come to the middle ear if small amounts of water make their way into the external auditory canal – but much harm **can** come to a child if he or she cannot swim. It is wise, however, to ban such activities as diving under water if grommets are in position in a child's ears.

Hearing aids, as a temporary measure, have gained popularity in recent years for the treatment of secretory otitis media. (See 'deafness'.)

THE FUTURE

Unless treatment for an acute attack of otitis media has been delayed or inadequate, or secretory otitis media has remained undiagnosed, most children will have normal hearing and few subsequent attacks of earache by the time they are 7 or 8 years of age.

Perthes' disease

Alternative names

Legge–Calve–Perthes' disease.
Coxa magna.
Osteochondritis.

INCIDENCE

Exact figures for this condition are not known, but it is thought that around 1 in every 2000 children is affected. Perthes' disease occurs in the 2–12-year age group, but most cases are seen between the ages of 4 and 8 years. Boys are about four times more frequently affected than are girls. A few of the children with Perthes' disease have the condition in both hips. Whilst there is no discernible genetic link, brothers and sisters of sufferers have a slightly higher chance of having the condition than does the general childhood population.

CAUSATION

Exactly why this condition should occur is uncertain. A temporary diminution in the blood supply to the head of the femur or thigh bone (the 'ball' of the 'ball-and-socket' hip joint) is the most probable cause. This and the compression exerted on this weight-bearing joint are thought to be the two aetiological factors.

In addition to bony changes there is swelling of the surrounding soft tissues. These two factors eventually lead to destruction of the normal anatomy of the joint. It is these changes that give rise to the typical characteristics of the condition.

CHARACTERISTICS

Limp: any child with a limp which lasts for longer than a few days should be investigated thoroughly. Obvious causes, such as a wound or a blister on the foot, can be easily eliminated. A limp, associated with an unusual lurching type of gait, can be one of the first signs of Perthes' disease – even before the child complains of pain.

Pain: this can either be felt in the affected joint itself or referred down the thigh into the knee. This pain can vary in intensity from day to day, although it is usually consistently worse after exercise. (Strangely enough, the degree of pain seems to bear little relationship to the changes seen on X-ray. So it is important that even a mild degree of pain should be thoroughly investigated.)

On examination of the leg there is found to be a **limitation of movement** of the hip. This is due to muscle spasm in an effort to protect the joint. The child will also actively dislike attempts to move the hip joint.

There is rarely any severe constitutional upset with Perthes' disease.

INVESTIGATIONS

X-ray of the affected joint will allow a definitive diagnosis, as the changes seen are quite typical of the condition. The space between the head of the thigh bone and the pelvis is seen to be wider than usual. This is due to the swelling of the surrounding soft tissues. With advanced disease, the usual smooth surface of the 'ball' of the hip joint is seen to be irregular and maybe to contain cysts. It is when the actual growing part of the bone is affected that permanent damage – such as shortening of the affected leg – can occur.

Following treatment, regular X-rays, at about 3-monthly intervals, are necessary to review progress. The hip joint will eventually heal and recalcify. The degree of residual disability will depend on the amount of bony destruction that has occurred during the active stages of the disease.

MANAGEMENT

In the initial stages of the disease, **bed rest** with the affected leg in **traction** is necessary. The leg is held in an immobile raised position to allow the hip to heal without the stresses and strains on the joint which inevitably occur when the child is walking or running.

Physiotherapy is vital during this stage to ensure that the muscles in the legs do not become weak during this period of inactivity.

Analgesics of appropriate type and dosage depending on the child's age and weight should be given if pain is severe.

Schooling for those children with Perthes' disease of school age will need to be kept up to date due to the unavoidable absences from school during treatment. Contact with the child's school can often be arranged, with appropriate work and activities sent to the child. This will obviate much of the boredom and frustration of enforced inactivity as well as keeping the young patient in touch with events at school.

Depending on the stage of the disease as seen on X-ray, the hip can eventually be immobilized in a special type of **splint** with the leg held outwards and rotated inwards. This is an incredibly awkward position, but it is surprising how quickly children adapt to this, and how mobile they become. With some rearrangements in the classroom and a sympathetic teacher, the child can once again attend school. This form of immobilization will need to be continued for several months.

Time off from school will be necessary for continuing **physiotherapy** to ensure that unused muscles do not become weak. Again, sympathetic understanding on the part of the child's teacher is vital.

Emotional support of both parents and child will be necessary during this long period of immobilization of the affected leg. Encouragement, from orthopaedic consultant, general practitioner, health visitor and school, can do much to help.

THE FUTURE

Depending on the severity of the Perthes' disease there may be, in a few children, some **shortening** of the leg on the affected side. This will only occur if the actual growing part of the bone has been affected. Usually, little effect is noticed even if this has occurred. In later adult life, **osteo-arthritis** in the affected hip may occur earlier in life than is usual following Perthes' disease in childhood.

SELF-HELP GROUP

Perthes' Association
42 Woodlands Road
Guildford
Surrey GU1 1RW
(Tel: 0483 306637)

OTHER TYPES OF OSTEOCHONDRITES

Osteochondritis is not confined to the hip joint. Other joints, and particular parts of bones, can also be affected. The disease process is exactly the same as that which causes Perthes' disease. These osteochondrites are given different names according to the bone affected.

Osgood–Schlatter's disease

This is an osteochondritis of the tibial tubercle – the small bony projection in the shin bone just below the knee.

Osgood–Schlatter's disease usually occurs in boys around the time of puberty. There is a painful swelling in this position on the leg, causing the boy to walk with a limp. X-ray changes are similar to those seen in Perthes' disease.

Treatment is by immobilization in plaster for 6–8 weeks, or temporary restriction of vigorous activity in mild cases. Following this, a gradual return to full activity, over the succeeding 2 months, is advisable. The help of a physiotherapist is valuable in strengthening muscles weakened by inactivity.

Sever's disease

This time it is the heel bone which is involved. Again, X-ray changes are similar, and the child will find walking painful. Once again, this condition occurs more commonly in adolescence. A walking plaster may be necessary for around 6 weeks to relieve pain, although fitting a raised heel to the shoe can sometimes give sufficient relief.

Kohler's disease

A small bone in the foot is the site of the osteochondritis in Kohler's disease. Boys between the ages of 3 and 8 years are most commonly affected. Again, a limp, with local pain and tenderness in the foot, are the symptoms of Kohler's disease. Walking tends to aggravate the pain.

A 6–8-week period of immobilization in a walking plaster will promote recovery.

All the above conditions heal readily, and leave no permanent after-effects.

Pityriasis

INCIDENCE

Pityriasis rosea (pityriasis alba is a similar condition, but is rarely seen) is an uncommon condition, but can give rise to much concern due to the extensive rash which is the main feature of the disease. Older children – over the age of 10 years – are the most usual sufferers. Pityriasis is frequently found during adolescence.

Both sexes are equally affected. Some authorities say that one attack of pityriasis confers immunity for life, but this is by no means necessarily so.

HISTORY

Pityriasis has been recognized for centuries. Pityriasis is a word derived from the Greek meaning 'bran'. This aptly describes the flaky scales on the skin which are the characteristics of the condition.

CAUSATION

Strangely enough, the exact cause of pityriasis is not clearly known. Various ideas have had their vogue, and range from a fungal infection, through an allergic manifestation to a viral origin. It is now thought that the last of these is the true cause, although no specific virus has so far been isolated.

Cases of pityriasis tend to occur in clusters. This adds extra force to the infective theory.

CHARACTERISTICS

Characteristically, pityriasis begins with one lesion on the skin, known as the **herald patch**. This is a single round eruption occurring anywhere on the body, but most usually on the chest, back or upper limbs. This patch can be anything up to 10 cm in diameter, and has a typical scaly appearance, often with a patch of clear skin in the centre. (If seen alone, this can easily be confused with a patch of discoid eczema.)

Within a week or two an **extensive rash** develops all over the body. Fortunately, hands, feet and face are usually spared, although the rash does occasionally extend to these exposed sites of the body. More of the rash tends to appear every 2 or 3 days for around 1 week. This rapidity of spread can be quite alarming, particularly in the skin-conscious adolescent. The rash may be **irritant**, but this is not always the case.

The rash will gradually disappear, but it will be between 3 and 8 weeks before the skin is finally completely clear – again a source of much distress. As with the herald patch, the lesions will clear initially in the centres, leaving a ruff of bran-like scales around the edges of the spots. Eventually the rash will disappear completely, leaving no residual trace of the once extensive eruptions.

Very occasionally, there may be a mild **fever** and a general feeling of **ill-health** before the rash becomes apparent, but this is unusual.

MANAGEMENT

There is little that can be done to speed the cure of this trivial, but nevertheless distressing, condition. If irritation is a problem, a **steroid cream** can be helpful, or an antihistamine given at night.

Reassurance that, within a few weeks, the rash will completely disappear is important. As mentioned previously, recurrence is rare, but can occur – often many years later.

There is no need for children with pityriasis to stay away from **school**, although it is important that teachers – and other parents – are reassured that the extensive rash is not infectious.

THE FUTURE

There are no adverse effects following an attack of pityriasis rosea.

Psoriasis

INCIDENCE

Psoriasis is known world-wide. It is usually thought of as a disease of adult life, but can, in fact, occur in the youngest of children. In babies a particular type of nappy-rash, which is very resistant to the usual forms of treatment, is thought to be often due to psoriasis.

Both sexes can be affected, girls more often than boys. There is often a strong family history of the condition.

HISTORY

It is possible that some of the leprose lesions described in antiquity may have been due to psoriasis.

CAUSATION

Psoriasis is considered to be a dominantly inherited disorder. If one parent has the condition, one out of four of the children will stand a chance of inheriting the disease. (Regretfully there is no way of predicting which child will be affected. Similarly if, for example, the first child in the family has psoriasis, this does not mean that the next three children will be free of the condition. The chances are one in four for each successive child.)

Faults in immunological function and also hormonal imbalance are thought to be implicated in psoriasis.

The onset of psoriasis frequently occurs following a bout of infection or any other form of stress such as, for example, an accident or a bereavement.

CHARACTERISTICS

In children, psoriasis usually begins in a slightly different form to the lesions seen in the adult form of the disease. The **rash** consists of small patches, or 'drops' (the name guttate psoriasis – 'gutta' meaning a 'drop' in Latin – is applied to these early lesions). They can occur anywhere on the body, including the face.

As the child matures, the rash changes its characteristics to those of the more adult form. This consists of larger plaques, with a white, scaly surface, mainly on knees, elbows and in the scalp.

In children, the rash of psoriasis is often preceded by an **upper respiratory tract infection** with streptococcal bacteria.

When psoriasis affects armpits, groins or the napkin area in babies, the scaliness is less in evidence and the rash is red and angry-looking. Typically, the edges of the rash of psoriasis have well-defined margins. The rash does not itch.

Psoriasis is a condition that fluctuates in **severity** throughout life. Periods of stress or infection will often increase the amount of rash seen.

Psoriasis is not an **infectious** condition, and this should be explained fully to parents and teachers as well as to the children themselves.

MANAGEMENT

Psoriasis is a skin condition for which there is no complete cure. But much improvement can be gained by the various forms of treatment available. It is important that both child and parent should understand this so that disappointment is not too great when the rash recurs. **Encouragement** to persevere with treatment and **emotional support** are vital as the child matures and learns to live with the inherited skin condition.

Sunlight usually has a beneficial effect on psoriasis. So children and adolescents should be encouraged to expose arms and legs with a psoriasis rash in summer time rather than covering up the scaly lesions in an attempt to hide them from their contemporaries.

Preparations in the form of ointments or pastes – based on tar and salicylic acid – are the most suitable for use with children. There are a wide range of these preparations and testing will decide which one is of the most benefit to each individual child.

Weak **steroid** preparations are also useful. These should be used for a short time only, due to the possible side-effects that can occur with these drugs. Unfortunately, there is often a relapse once these preparations are withdrawn.

If the child has an upper respiratory tract infection at a time when the rash is at its worst, a course of **penicillin** will often clear the rash as well as curing the respiratory tract infection.

Long-term follow-up of children with this unpleasant condition is important, preferably by the same doctor, who will be able to reassure and encourage, knowing the previous condition of the child's skin.

Children with psoriasis can suffer from taunts at **school**. This will require sympathetic handling by teachers, who should be informed of the non-infectious – and also recurrent – nature of the condition.

Certain **careers** will be inadvisable for children with psoriasis. They should be advised against considering careers such as those in chemistry, beauty therapy or certain artistic activities when the time comes for choices to be made.

COMPLICATIONS

Psoriasis is regretfully a life-long condition which is characterized by periods of remission and relapse. Treatment will need to be varied according to the position and severity of the lesions at any one time.

SELF-HELP GROUP

The Psoriasis Association
7 Milton Street
Northampton NN2 7JG
(Tel. 0604 711129)

Rubella

Alternative name

German measles.

INCIDENCE

The true incidence of rubella is exceedingly difficult to determine, as many of these infections are so mild as to pass unnoticed. From studies on antibody levels against the infection in adult populations it is thought that around 90% of town-dwellers have suffered from an attack of rubella in their youth – many of them probably without realizing this. People who live in more rural areas have a lower incidence due to their decreased likelihood of meeting the infection. It seems that rubella is primarily a disease of childhood, the infection most probably being acquired between the ages of 5 and 12 years – the primary school years. Rubella has been a notifiable disease since 1988.

HISTORY

Rubella has been known for many years. The rather unfortunate name of 'German measles' arose from the early descriptions of the infection in Germany, and from a slight, superficial resemblance to measles. In fact, the infection is no more common in Germany than anywhere else, and certainly has no relationship at all to measles!

It was only in 1962 that the rubella virus was finally identified and cultured – surprisingly late for so common a disease.

The importance of this mild disease lies in the devastating effects it can have on the unborn baby if the mother contracts the infection during the first 3 months of pregnancy. These effects were discovered, through brilliant 'detective work', by an Australian doctor in the 1960s.

CAUSATION

Rubella is caused by a virus. The incubation period of the infection is between 14 and 21 days.

CHARACTERISTICS

The typical **rash** is often the first sign of the disease in children. This begins on the face, and rapidly spreads over the chest, back and, to a lesser extent, the limbs. The rash is fine and pink, with the spots in some cases becoming so extensive that they coalesce.

The length of time for which the rash persists is very variable. It is usually apparent for anything up to 5 days, but can occasionally be so transient as to not be seen at all or to last merely a few hours.

Swelling of the **lymph glands** in the neck is a constant feature of infection with the rubella virus. This enlargement can precede the appearance of the rash. The swollen glands can be tender, particularly the ones at the back of the neck. In fact tenderness on combing a child's hair is often the first clue that a rubella infection is present.

Mild **fever**, **headache** and general **malaise** can accompany the infection but frequently the child may not feel any ill-effects from the disease.

MANAGEMENT

There is no specific treatment for an attack of rubella, and, indeed, this is rarely required due to the mild nature of the disease.

Analgesics may be necessary for headache and fever control, in appropriate dosage and type for the individual child. (Do remember that aspirin compound should not be used for children under the age of 12 years, due to the possibility of Reye's syndrome.)

Children should be kept away from **school** during the acute stage of the disease when the rash is in evidence or they are feeling unwell. With a fleeting rash and a mild infection this can be difficult to implement. But if there is any suggestion that a child may have rubella the school should be informed. Any pregnant teacher can then take steps to determine her immunity – or otherwise – to rubella, if this has not already been done.

COMPLICATIONS

Rubella has a very low complication rate. A transient **arthritis** can occur in the small joints of the body – hands, wrists and ankles in particular. This occurs more frequently with adults suffering from the disease, but can also occur in children.

Encephalitis (inflammation of the brain) can occur following rubella, but is very rare.

Epistaxis (nose bleeding), **haematuria** (blood in the urine) or **purpura** (small bleeding spots under the skin) can also occur in association with an attack of rubella, due to changes in the blood as a result of the infection. This will resolve without specific treatment.

PREVENTION

Rubella is a disease preventable by immunization. It is important that the highest levels of protection by immunization are reached in order to reduce to a minimum the number of babies born with the 'rubella syndrome'. This is a devastating condition in which babies can be born deaf, blind and/or with a heart condition if their mothers have contracted rubella during the first 3 months of their pregnancy. Ensuring that the pool of infection amongst young children is reduced lowers the likelihood of rubella being a possibility at this time in a normal reproductive life.

Until 1988, all schoolgirls in Britain were offered immunization against rubella at 10–14 years of age in order to protect them during the critical child-bearing years. Since this date, however, immunization against rubella has been given, as part of the MMR (measles, mumps and rubella) injection, between the ages of 1 and 2 years.

Rubella immunization will still be available to girls between 10 and 14 years of age, and also to those women who on blood testing are found to be non-immune to rubella, for the foreseeable future. This will continue until the 'catch-up' time, when all babies have had this immunization routinely, arrives.

THE FUTURE

There are virtually no long-term effects following an attack of rubella, apart from the possible effects on the fetus if rubella is contracted during pregnancy. It is to be hoped that a time can be visualized when no further rubella syndrome babies are born, due to the elimination of this particular infection.

Scabies

INCIDENCE

Scabies is an infestation with a mite. It occurs world-wide and is especially common in underdeveloped countries of the world, and also in places where hygiene is less than perfect. Scabies is unusual in that there appear to be wide fluctuations in incidence. Epidemics seem to arise about every 15 years or so. In recent years the incidence of scabies has markedly increased. These facts are possibly due to a form of natural immunity to the mite which develops amongst communities. The recent higher reported incidence indicates that this immunity may be on the decline.

January, April and November, for some obscure reason, are the months in Britain when most cases occur.

HISTORY

Scabies has been known since the seventeenth century. It is said to be the first disease in man to have a known cause – that is, infestation with the mite *Sarcoptes scabies*.

CAUSATION

Infestation with a specific mite is the cause of the symptoms. The adult female scabies mite is only around 0.5 mm long, and has been graphically described as closely resembling a minute tortoise. This female burrows into the skin by initially standing on her head to gain entry, and then burrowing along parallel to the skin surface. As she travels along, eggs are laid. These burrowing activities leave S-shaped tracks which are visible to the naked eye, and are typical of the condition. It can be difficult to see the tracks as they are so small and are also frequently overlaid with skin inflammation due to scratching.

CHARACTERISTICS

Scabies is characterized by intense **itching**. This is worse at night when the body is warm. The irritation not only occurs in the positions where the mite is active, but can occur all over the body. This is thought to be due to a generalized hypersensitivity to the presence of the mite. The **rash** associated with scabies is very variable. For example, raised blistery spots can be seen alongside raised red discrete spots all overlaid with scratch marks caused by an attempt to quell the overwhelming irritation. Also, as a result of this scratching, the skin can become infected.

With all these various lesions on the skin it can often be very difficult to find the 'burrows' of the scabies mite which are the basic cause of all the problems.

The most usual **sites** for scabies to occur are around the insides of the wrists, under the arms, between the fingers and around those areas of the body where clothes fit tightly, such as the waist and groin. Other areas of the body can also show signs of the infestation, but usually the palms of the hands, the soles of the feet and the face and scalp regions remain clear. (One exception to this latter fact is when the infestation occurs in young babies. In these infants, the face and hands are often also affected.)

The diagnosis of scabies is often delayed due to the difficulty of finding the typical burrows of the scabies mite amongst all the possible differing lesions on the skin. The marked irritation should cause suspicion, especially if more than one member of the family – or nursery/school class – is having this problem.

The infestation is passed on from person to person by close physical contact. Scabies cannot be 'caught' from clothing or bedding.

MANAGEMENT

There are a number of preparations available with which to treat scabies. Benzyl benzoate emulsion is probably the most well known and effective. This emulsion should be applied to the whole of the child's body with the exception of the head and neck. It should be applied following a warm bath and allowed to dry on the body. Treatment should be given on two consecutive nights to ensure that all the mites – in all stages of development – are eradicated. If there is a good deal of secondary infection as a result of frequent and persistant scratching – which can be almost impossible to control – an appropriate **antibiotic** will need to be prescribed. The **whole family** may need to be treated if there is any suggestion that they too are affected by the presence of a rash and persistent irritation.

An unfortunate manifestation of scabies is that even though adequate treatment has been carried out the **itch** may still persist for several weeks. A specific cream is available which will help to control this unpleasant aspect of the condition.

Nightwear and **bed-linen** will need to be laundered in the usual way following treatment with benzyl benzoate in order to remove the unpleasant odour.

Schooling can continue as usual once the treatment has been undertaken.

Scarlet fever

INCIDENCE

The exact incidence of scarlet fever is not known, but the infection is certainly far less in evidence than 50 years ago. At this time, scarlet fever was a much-dreaded disease, both from the point of view of the severity of the illness and because of the possible complications – rheumatic fever and glomerulonephritis. These complications were frequently seen due to the absence of any specific treatment for scarlet fever.

Also, over the years the virulence of the bacteria causing this infection appears to have diminished, again making the disease less serious when it does occur.

Scarlet fever is an uncommon condition in the pre-school child.

HISTORY

Between the two World Wars, fever, or isolation, hospitals were an integral part of the health scene. Patients, both children and adults, were nursed in these isolation units in an attempt to control the spread of the infections. Before the advent of antibiotics, isolation of the sufferers had a large part to play in the control of infectious disease. Scarlet fever patients formed a large part of the inmates of these fever hospitals. Today, antibiotic treatment has replaced the need for such isolation facilities.

CAUSATION

Scarlet fever is caused by a particular strain of the group A beta-haemolytic streptococcal bacteria. (Beta-haemolytic streptococcal bacteria are classified according to the changes seen when the bacteria are grown under laboratory conditions.) These bacteria are also one of the organisms that are the cause of the skin infection impetigo.

The bacteria are usually passed on from child to child by droplet infection. They can also be passed on via a wound, burn or skin infection contaminated with the particular bacteria.

The incubation period is a short one. One to seven days is quoted, but 3–4 days is the more usual time at which symptoms appear after contact with a sufferer.

CHARACTERISTICS

Scarlet fever usually starts very abruptly with the sudden onset of:

- **headache**;
- **very sore throat**;
- **fever**, which can be very high for the first few days of the illness;
- **vomiting**.

These features can also be seen at the onset of any severe throat infection or tonsillitis. It is when the typical **rash** of scarlet fever appears that a definite diagnosis can be made. This is usually on the second day of the illness. The rash is typically one of a generalized redness (or erythema) of the skin with specific small spots of an intense scarlet colour (hence the name of this condition). The rash begins on the face and rapidly spreads to the neck and chest and then on to the limbs. Armpits, elbow creases and groin all show a dense concentration of the rash. Also, the rash on the face is quite typical inasmuch as the area around the mouth is free of the bright red rash.

The rash starts to fade after 2 or 3 days. Following this, in severe cases, the skin where the rash has been at its height begins to peel off, leaving clear skin underneath. Mild attacks do not show this desquamation process. (In olden days this peeled skin was much feared, as it was thought to carry the infection. It is now recognized that the shed skin is sterile.)

With the disappearance of the rash the young patient will begin to feel better. The fever will drop, sore throat and headache will disappear and appetite will improve.

The **tonsils** and whole throat will be reddened with white patches covering the surface.

Ears can also be affected along with the generalized throat infection, and are seen to be reddened on examination.

The appearance of the **tongue** is quite unique in scarlet fever. Initially it is coated with a white, fur-like substance with the bright red spots of the infection showing through. At this stage it is termed the 'white strawberry' tongue! In a couple of days the whole tongue becomes red – the 'red strawberry' tongue.

INVESTIGATIONS

Throat swabs can be taken and sent to the laboratory for the infective organism to be determined if the diagnosis is uncertain. But this is rarely done as scarlet fever can so readily be diagnosed from the clinical signs and symptoms.

MANAGEMENT

Antibiotic treatment has transformed scarlet fever from a serious disease, with the possibility of long-term complications, to a relatively mild – although unpleasant – illness. Penicillin is the antibiotic usually prescribed to treat this infection, but erythromycin can also be used for children who are allergic to penicillin.

Within 48 hours of starting treatment there is no longer any possibility of passing on the infection to another member of the family.

It is important that the antibiotic treatment is continued for 10 days in order to completely eradicate the bacteria. There is no need to give penicillin as a prophylactic measure to other children in the family, unless they are taking steroids for some other condition. Under these circumstances they should be given penicillin to ensure that they do not suffer an attack from the streptococcal bacillus.

Analgesics – usually in the form of some paracetamol compound for children – can be given to relieve headache and sore throat. These drugs will also help to lower the temperature, and so will make the young patient feel more comfortable.

A light **diet** with plenty of cool **fluids** is helpful during the stage of the acute sore throat. The child will usually have little, or no, appetite for solid food, but it is important that adequate fluids should be given to prevent dehydration, which can occur, especially if the fever is high.

Bedrest for the first 2 or 3 days, when the temperature is at its height, will probably be most comfortable for the child. As soon as wishes to get up are expressed, quiet play in warm room is quite satisfactory.

Schooling can be resumed as soon as the child's general health and energy have returned to normal. This includes, of course, the complete disappearance of the rash, no further sore throat and a return to normal appetite and interest in usual activities.

COMPLICATIONS

With immediate and adequate treatment with penicllin, or other appropriate drug, these are uncommon.

Acute otitis media, in which there are earache and redness on examination of the eardrum, can occur as part of the initial symptomatology. The penicillin will rapidly cure this possible complication.

Sinusitis, and/or enlarged neck glands, can also occur following scarlet fever.

In the pre-antibiotic era, **glomerulonephritis** often occurred a few weeks or months following the primary illness. In this condition, the kidneys can be seriously damaged and leave the sufferer with long-term problems. This rarely, if ever, happens today.

Similarly, **rheumatic fever**, which frequently affected the heart, was a feared complication of scarlet fever. Again, this is virtually unknown today.

Bronchopneumonia was again a common complication. But antibiotics ensure that this rarely happens nowadays.

PREVENTION

There is no immunization available against scarlet fever. The causative organism, the streptococcal bacterium, is to be found in the throats of 10–20% perfectly fit children. With such a widespread occurrence, immunization would be difficult and as the treatment is so relatively easy and successful, there would not seem to be the need for a vaccine. Early diagnosis and treatment are the mainstays to prevent the serious complications of the disease.

THE FUTURE

An attack of scarlet fever, as discussed above, rarely leads to any long-term complications these days. One attack does not necessarily lead to immunity from acquiring a sore throat with the streptococcal bacterium as the causative organism, but scarlet fever itself rarely occurs more than once.

Squint

Alternative name

Strabismus.

INCIDENCE

Whilst squints in children are not a disease entity in the same way as, for example, are an infectious condition or a congenital problem, early treatment is vital if full vision is to be preserved.

The exact incidence of squints in children is not documented. But it is thought that around 50% of children who do have a squint have someone else in the family who has the same condition. The squint itself is not directly inherited, but the factors which are associated with the production of the squint can be passed on from generation to generation. In view of this, it is important that the brothers and sisters of a child with a squint should also be examined for this condition.

It is especially important to diagnose those children in whom the squint is not immediately obvious. Small or latent squints can have as great a deleterious effect on good binocular vision as can a more obvious squint.

Squints can occur in any axis of the eye. But by far the commonest types of squint are the convergent type (in which one eye is seen to turn inwards) and the divergent type (in which one eye is seen to turn outwards).

All babies squint at times for the first few weeks after birth before muscle co-ordination is fully developed. But any squint in a baby over the age of 4 months should be investigated.

CAUSATION

There are a number of conditions which can be factors in the aetiology of a squint, as follows.

- A **refractive error** in one eye is by far the commonest cause of a squint. Under these circumstances one eye focuses clearly on an object at a different distance from that of the other eye. For example, a convergent squint can occur when one eye focuses more clearly on an object at a greater distance away than does the other eye. (This is known as hypermetropia.) To pull these two perceived objects into one image the 'long-distance'-seeing eye will need to accommodate (pulled by the eye muscles into the right position) to a greater extent than the other eye. Conversely, a short-sighted (myopic) eye – focusing clearly on nearer objects – will need less accommodation, and so a divergent squint will be the result.
- **Injuries** to the cornea resulting in scarring of this external sensitive part of the eye can also give rise to a squint. This has a similar effect to that produced by a short-sighted eye, inasmuch as vision in the damaged eye is reduced.
- The onset of a squint in a previously non-squinting child can also be the first clue to **disease** of the **retina** or **optic nerve** such as, for example, a retinoblastoma.
- **Occlusion** of one eye by a pad or bandage, following some injury to an eye or the face, can cause a squint to develop in a surprisingly short time. The covered eye will become non-seeing or 'amblyopic' due to disuse. Treatment to reverse this process must be undertaken with a degree of urgency to prevent permanent loss of vision in this eye.

Whilst a simple refractive error is the commonest cause of a squint, the other possible factors must always be borne in mind.

CHARACTERISTICS

Squints, as mentioned previously, come in a variety of guises – **convergent** or **divergent** and also, to a much lesser extent, in the vertical axis. Children with squints in the vertical axis will often tilt their heads to compensate for the squint – a useful clue that a squint may be present, although not immediately obvious.

As well as these differences in direction, squints can be alternating in character – that is, one eye being fixed on an object at one time only to be quickly followed by the other eye being fixed on the object instead. In this condition, true binocular vision (in which the two eyes fix and focus on one object to produce one image) is never achieved.

Squints can cause two images to be seen, although there is only one object (double vision). This is obviously not a situation which can continue! So the part of the brain concerned with vision will suppress one of these images – from the squinting eye, for example. As a knock-on result of this the eye will eventually lose all ability to see. This condition is known as 'amblyopia'.

It is to prevent this loss of vision in one eye that early intervention in squints is vital, as without treatment the lack of vision can become permanent.

Squints can be very obvious, even to the casual observer, or can be so small as to be virtually undetectable without special tests. It is important that observations by parents on their child's possible squint should not be dismissed, but investigated fully.

A 'pseudo-squint' is often seen in children who have especially marked folds of skin (epicanthic folds) over the near side of their eyes. These skin folds can give the appearance of a squint by obscuring more of the white of the eye on the inner side. Specific tests (see below) will differentiate this effect from true squints. This condition is more commonly noticed in younger children before the development of definite strong facial features.

Similar effects can also occur in children who have a broad bridge to their nose, or who have an asymmetrical face for some reason. Again, special tests will differentiate this.

A **latent squint** can become obvious when a child is ill with some concurrent infection. Muscle control at this time is imperfect and a squint can be clearly seen. On recovery the squint will disappear, but if this is noticed it is as well to check with an orthoptist that there is no squint.

(Note that squints are not caused by anxiety, fear or infectious disease, as some 'old wives' tales' would have one believe.)

INVESTIGATIONS

Test for **refractive errors**: these will include tests for short sight, long sight and astigmatism, with special reference to differences between the two eyes. (An astigmatism occurs when the lens of the eye is less than perfectly shaped, so that distorted images bounce off this ill-shaped refractive surface.)

Examination of **light reflexes**: shining a light, from a pencil torch, for example, into the child's eye will show whether or not the reflection from the light occurs in the same position in each eye. If, for example, the light is reflected to the right of the pupil in one eye and over the pupil in the other, some degree of squint is present.

The **cover test**: this test involves covering one of the child's eyes with a hand, or card, while the child is focusing on a distant object. On removal of the cover, the covered eye will be seen to move if a squint is present. If there is no squint neither eye will move on taking away the covering hand or card. This test should be repeated two or three times in quick succession.

Orthoptic tests, with special equipment, to measure the **angle** of the **squint** can be carried out once the presence of a definite squint has been established.

Full **examination** by an opthalmologist, with the eyes fully dilated, is necessary when causes other than simple refractive errors are suspected. This is vital to exclude serious eye disease.

MANAGEMENT

Correction of any refractive error is the first essential requirement. This involves routine tests, appropriate to the age of the child, for long or short sight as well as for an astigmatism. Spectacles are then prescribed to correct these errors. In many cases this will result in an improvement of the squint. It will be necessary to constantly review the strength of the visual correction. With growth the refractive errors in a long-sighted child can improve so much that the spectacles can be discarded at a later date.

Occlusion of the good eye for 1 or 2 weeks at a time may be required to obtain good vision in the squinting eye. This is often necessary if a degree of amblyopia has developed in the squinting eye.

Orthoptic exercises are also valuable in producing good binocular vision.

If the above treatments are not adequate, **surgery** can be necessary to correct the squint. This is carried out under a general anaesthetic. The muscles moving the eyes are then lengthened, shortened or repositioned according to the type and degree of the squint.

Occasionally, instillation of **eye-drops** which cause accommodation of the squinting eye to decrease have been used with success in small-angle squints.

Other, more recent and experimental, treatments have been used to induce a temporary, partial paralysis of the eye muscles. This allows time for binocular vision to become established.

THE FUTURE

Amblyopia: this condition is the result that can occur if a squint remains undiagnosed and untreated for some time. Amblyopia becomes of great importance to the person if, at a later date, vision is lost in the normally seeing eye. Full vision can then never be fully restored to an amblyopic eye.

SELF-HELP GROUPS

Royal National Institute for the Blind (RNIB)
224 Great Portland Street
London W1N 6AA
(Tel. 071 388 1266)

The Partially Sighted Society
62 Salusbury Road
London NW6 6NS
(Tel. 071 372 1551)

It is to be hoped that no child with a simple squint will ever need to be in contact with either of the above societies. Only if the squint is an early manifestation of some other ocular disease should severe visual handicap be a problem.

Threadworm

Alternative names

Pin worm.
Seat worm.

INCIDENCE

Threadworms are common throughout the world and are – surprisingly – especially common in countries with a colder climate. The age group most often affected is that between 5 and 9 years – the primary school years. (Research in the late 1980s suggested that there is a further peak in incidence between the ages of 30 and 49 years. Possibly this is the age group who most frequently live with children in the 5–9 year age group, and so are infected along with their children.)

Infestation occurs more commonly in urban areas. It is thought that up to 50% of London children are infested with threadworms at any one time.

CAUSATION

Infestation with threadworms is passed on from child to child by hand contact, or contact with soiled underclothes or bed-linen. The tiny eggs of the threadworm are laid, in many thousands, around the child's anus during sleep. These eggs can then be transferred on fingers, following scratching, to the mouth. The ingested eggs hatch on their way through the intestine. The adult worms then mate, the female again lays further thousands of eggs and the cycle is repeated. The eggs can survive in dust, at room temperature, for up to 2 or 3 weeks. (Domestic animals, of any kind, play no part in the dissemination of threadworms. This differs from the mode of spread of other worms.)

CHARACTERISTICS

Over the years, threadworms have been thought to cause many symptoms in children such as nail-biting, convulsions and hyperactivity to mention just a few. None of these conditions are in fact due to threadworms.

Irritation around the **anus** can be due to the presence of the worm.

It is also possible that **sleep** can be disturbed by the presence of the egg-laying worm. Some authorities also consider that **bed-wetting** can occur due to this cause.

In girls, **irritation** around the **vulval area** can result from infestation with threadworms.

Parents can also, at times, be alarmed to see worms in their child's stools. This does not occur, however, as frequently as may be expected due to the smallness of the worm – only around 10 mm long.

INVESTIGATIONS

The best method to determine whether or not a child is infested with threadworms is to wrap a piece of Sellotape (sticky side out) around a test tube or spatula and apply this to the child's anus. The tape is then transferred to a microscope slide. The eggs, if present, can then readily be seen when the slide is visualized under the microscope. (The child should not have bathed or had his or her bowels open before this test is performed.) It may be necessary to repeat this investigation for three consecutive days as the worms do not necessarily pass through the intestine in a regular manner.

MANAGEMENT

There are a number of **drugs** which will effectively eliminate threadworms. Usually only one dose is needed. It is advisable that all members of the family should be treated, due to the many thousands of eggs that can be present in the bed-linen and in the general household dust.

Hygiene, especially in personal cleanliness, is vital in controlling infestations with threadworms. Children should be taught the importance of **hand-washing** before meals and after visiting the toilet.

Fingernails should be cut short to reduce the possibility of the eggs remaining in this situation. Frequent changes of underwear and bed-linen are also of importance in the control of infestation with threadworms.

Parents will also need **reassurance** that they are not alone in having thread-worms as visitors to their family, and that their child will not suffer permanent harm.

COMPLICATIONS

Very occasionally there may be such a heavy infestation of threadworms in the bowel that the child may complain of **abdominal pain**. This will be cured by the appropriate treatment to eliminate the worms.

(Threadworms have been found in the lumen of the appendix following removal of this organ, but it is not thought that this has any bearing on the onset of the appendicitis.)

PREVENTION

This is limited to good personal hygiene and prompt and adequate treatment of the whole family if an infestation is found to be present.

Tics

Alternative names

Habit disorder.
Habit spasm.

INCIDENCE

It is thought that the rapid, repetitive, involuntary muscular movements known as habit spasms affect as many as 10% of the childhood population at any one time. Children between the ages of 7 and 12 years are most commonly affected. Boys outnumber girls by 3 to 1 in these habits.

There is frequently a family history of habit spasms. Some habit spasms do persist into adult life.

HISTORY

A variety of bizarre tics have been described in literature – Dickens being the master of this.

CAUSATION

Frequently a **stressful** home or school situation can be found with a child has a tic. It would seem likely that the tic has been developed almost as a superstitious ritual against the stress in these circumstances.

Imitation is also a powerful stimulus to the development of a tic. A schoolmate with twitchy eyes, or a grandfather with a limp, can often be found in the child's immediate environment. Differentiation of simple tics from chorea and the Gilles de la Tourette syndrome must be made.

In chorea (a symptom seen in a number of illnesses, including a type of cerebral palsy or following encephalitis for example) the movements are not so stereotyped and predictable as with habit spasms.

Gilles de la Tourette syndrome is a particularly distressing ailment where there are many, violent complex muscular tics associated frequently with the repetition of obscene words and an odd form of barking cough. This syndrome is extremely difficult to treat and can continue into adult life in around 50% of cases – a point of difference from common tics.

CHARACTERISTICS

Tics can affect any part of the body but are most usually seen to involve the head and neck areas. **Blinking** of the eyes, **twisting** of the mouth and/or **shrugging** of the shoulders are amongst the commonest tics noted.

It is always the **same group of muscles** involved in each series of movements, so that one is aware in advance of exactly what will be happening next. (This is in direct contrast to the involuntary movements due to other physical causes.)

Repetitive coughing, swallowing or sneezing are other irritating forms of tics found in children. These tics often begin under circumstances of acute embarrassment for the child, and continue when the particular stress is removed.

MANAGEMENT

Most cases of habit spasm resolve spontaneously given time. But it is thought that about 6% of children with tics will still have their specific habit spasm when adult.

Parents should be advised not to **grumble at** or **ridicule** their child with a tic. This is counterproductive and only draws attention to the problem.

Family therapy can help where there are family tensions and anxieties. General practitioners will be able to give advice on where and how to contact skilled people to undertake this therapy.

Behaviour therapy is also helpful. Therapists can help parents with techniques to distract the child's attention when the tic is manifest.

Tranquillizers are a last resort to be tried, particularly if the child is over-active in addition to having a tic. These drugs must be carefully controlled, however, and never continued for any length of time.

THE FUTURE

The majority of simple tics resolve themselves by the time the teenage years are reached. A few adults will still have their tics in evidence throughout their lives, and these will become part of their individual personalities.

Tics caused by chorea or the Gilles de la Tourette syndrome have a less successful outcome and need specialized treatment.

SELF-HELP GROUP

There is a specific self-help group for parents of children with the Gilles de la Tourette syndrome:

Tourette Syndrome (UK) Association
Valley Mead
27 Monkton Street
Ryde
Isle of Wight PO33 2BY

Tonsillitis

INCIDENCE

As tonsillitis is not a notifiable condition, there are no figures available for this unpleasant infection of the throat so common in children. But all doctors' surgeries – especially during the winter months – will see several children every week with tonsillitis.

Pre-school and early school-age children will usually suffer from around three to four upper respiratory infections during the course of any one year. Whilst all these infections are by no means tonsillitis, a significant number will involve the pads of lymphatic tissue known as the tonsils – the 'watch-dogs' of the throat.

(Anatomically the pharynx, housing the tonsils at either side, is closely allied to the middle ear. Infection frequently occurs in both these parts of the body simultaneously – but for descriptive purposes it is best that they are discussed separately.)

Boys and girls are affected equally, and tonsillitis is seen world-wide.

CAUSATION

The tonsils are two masses of lymphoid tissue situated at the back of the throat, and in children they are relatively large up to the age of 8 years – even when clear of infection. They fulfil the function of dealing with bacteria and viruses before these invaders have the chance to proceed to the lower respiratory tract – the lungs and associated structures. As the tonsils perform their work dealing with infection, they become red and swollen. During this process, pain is felt and there is also a generalized constitutional upset.

Tonsillitis can be caused by either bacteria or viruses. It is impossible to determine which infecting organism is causing the symptoms without laboratory confirmation from a swab of the child's throat.

CHARACTERISTICS

Fever is one of the first and most common signs of tonsillitis. In young children in particular this can be high, and can give rise to **febrile convulsions**.

(These are convulsions caused by the reaction of the immature brain to a high body temperature. They rarely occur after the age of 5 years.)

A **sore throat** is more often complained of by older children than those in the under-5 bracket. These latter children frequently complain of a '**tummy-ache**' rather than a sore throat. In both age groups there will be a **reluctance to eat**.

On looking down the throat of the sufferer, the cause of the problem will become obvious. The tonsils are **red and swollen**. In really severe infections, the two tonsils are seen to almost meet in the mid-line of the throat – causing no surprise that the child is refusing food!

Swollen glands in the neck are also a frequent feature of tonsillitis. These cervical glands drain infection from the back of the throat, and in so doing become enlarged and tender.

A **blocked, stuffy nose** can also accompany an infection in the tonsils. This is due to associated infection in the adenoids – masses of lymphoid tissue situated at the back of the nose. These tissues also become swollen and inflamed by the infective process.

The child with tonsillitis will feel generally **unwell** and miserable.

INVESTIGATIONS

Tonsillitis is diagnosed by the clinical signs and symptoms. Theoretically a throat swab sent to the laboratory will determine the causative infective organism. In practice this is rarely done, as treatment needs to be started before the laboratory results become available.

MANAGEMENT

The acute attack

Penicillin is the antibiotic of first choice for an attack of tonsillitis, and will relieve unpleasant symptoms within 24–48 hours. It is important, however, that the full course that has been prescribed is taken, in order to fully eradicate the invading organism.

Paracetamol (in doses and strengths appropriate to the age of the child) should be given – at 4-hourly intervals if necessary initially – to relieve sore throat and headache. This drug will also help to lower the temperature.

Fluids only for the first 24–48 hours of the infection will be all that the young sufferer will be willing to take. It is vital that sufficient fluid is given at this time. Children can quickly become dehydrated due to the high fever so frequently seen during an acute attack of tonsillitis.

Bed rest is not essential, unless the child feels more comfortable tucked up in bed. Quiet play in a warm room with the chance to lie down on occasions is usually a favoured option for a young child with an acute attack of tonsillitis.

Tonsillectomy: this operation has had its fashions – tonsils being very readily removed for the slightest reason in bygone days. Today's criteria for this operation are more rigid. Most ear, nose and throat surgeons would only consider removing a child's tonsils if:

- the child has suffered from more than three attacks of confirmed tonsillitis in 1 year over a 2-year period; and/or
- the tonsils are so large as to meet in the mid-line even when an acute infection is not present – this state of affairs can be dangerous to normal breathing, especially during sleep.

Tonsillectomy is performed by an ear, nose and throat surgeon under a general anaesthetic. At the time the surgeon will also consider whether or not removal of the adenoids is necessary. A stay of one or two nights in hospital is the general rule.

Children recover very quickly from the removal of their tonsils – far more rapidly than do adults undergoing this procedure. Cool fluids and a soft easy-to-swallow diet for a day or two are all that are needed by way of post-operative care.

For school-age children, a couple of weeks off school is advisable to ensure that further throat infections are not contracted too soon after the operation.

THE FUTURE

If a child's tonsils have been chronically infected for a number of years with frequent attacks of acute infection, he or she will be seen to benefit enormously from tonsillectomy. Appetite, energy and general wellbeing will all improve and growth will often show a spurt.

On the downside, however, the mere fact of having had a tonsillectomy does not mean that sore throats are a thing of the past! Throat infections can – and do – still occur. But these are less frequent and recovery is quicker in the child whose tonsils had been a source of chronic infection.

Toxocara

INCIDENCE

The incidence of infections with toxocara – a type of roundworm – is not precisely known. Infections with this parasite may be more than is recognized, the child's immunity being built up before the condition is diagnosed.

CAUSATION

The toxocara canis worm is a normal inhabitant of the intestine of the young dog and the fox. These animals gain natural immunity to the parasite by around 6 months of age, and the adult worms are then expelled from their bodies at this time – so no ill-effects are seen in older dogs. But during pregnancy, bitches lose this immunity. Reinfection, or reactivation of the dormant larvae, occurs, thereby affecting the unborn puppies. So, at birth, these puppies are infected with the toxocara worm.

Children acquire the infection by swallowing the minute eggs of the toxocara – acquiring these either directly from the tongues of the puppies when they are licked, or from crawling around on carpets, lawns and other areas where eggs may be deposited. As would be expected, younger children – during the crawling years especially – comprise the most frequently affected age group. At this age, too, exploration of everyday objects is largely done by taking them to the mouth.

When inside the child's body the larvae (arising from the ingested eggs) have difficulty in finding their way to the intestine – where, in the dog and fox, they normally find their home. So they wander aimlessly around the body, setting up areas of inflammation in a variety of sites in the child's body – kidneys, lungs, muscles, brain and eyes can all be possibly affected. (This wandering is known by the splendidly descriptive name of 'visceral larvae migrans'.)

It is thought that the type of toxocara affecting cats – toxocara catis – can also cause similar symptoms.

CHARACTERISTICS

Signs and symptoms of infection with toxocara can be very diverse. The diagnosis of infection with toxocara may never be made as there are such a wide variety of possible non-specific symptoms, and the child may recover spontaneously. However, certain clues can help, as follows.

- The age of the child affected is usually between 1 and 7 years – the early years of crawling and putting many different objects into the mouth. At this age, also, hygiene is rudimentary!
- There is frequently the arrival in the home of a new puppy prior to the onset of symptoms.

Signs and symptoms of infection can include:

- **failure to thrive adequately** – for example, poor weight gain and lack of general growth;
- a liking of eating all kinds of strange substances, such as earth and coal – this is known as **pica**;
- a low-grade **fever**;
- a **cough**, with episodes of wheezing;
- **anaemia**;
- **convulsions**;
- **blurring** of vision with possible subsequent loss of vision due to involvement of the retina.

The blurring is caused by inflammation of this vital part of the eye, and the possible subsequent loss of vision is caused by the detachment of the retina. Children with these ocular manifestations of toxocara tend to be in the older age group – between 7 and 9 years. Not all these symptoms, of course, occur in any one infected child. The symptoms will depend on which organ, or system of the body, is involved in the infection.

Untreated, the infection runs a slow, benign course with the child's natural defence mechanisms eventually overcoming the infection. Usually within 18 months, full health is restored.

INVESTIGATIONS

Blood tests will show if any **anaemia** is present, and can also be used for serological testing to determine if antibodies against toxocara are present. (It is interesting to note that up to 7% of adults show positive results to this latter test. This implies that they have been infected, at some time or other in their earlier life, by toxocara. No very obvious symptoms may have occurred – that can be remembered – but they have successfully overcome the infection.)

MANAGEMENT

Often the diagnosis of toxocara is uncertain for some time and the child's very general and non-specific symptoms are treated empirically. For example, antibiotics are given for the cough, and iron medication for the anaemia. These medicines will result in improvement in the child's general health, as there can be added infection in the respiratory tract, and an iron-deficient anaemia as a result of a poor appetite.

Once investigations have proved that infection with toxocara is present, there are several specific drugs that can be used with success, although treatment may take several weeks. Steroids can also be used to advantage to reduce the inflammation at various sites in the body.

COMPLICATIONS

The most serious is the loss of vision which can result from the larvae migrating to the eye. Again, there are specific drugs available which are valuable in treating this condition, and can help to preserve vision.

PREVENTION

Infection of children with toxocara has evoked much 'anti-dog' publicity over recent years. But two points must be remembered, as follows.

1. Infections of all kinds abound in our immediate environs and toxocara is just one of them. With care and good hygiene this infection can be contained as readily – or more so – than many others.
2. Pets of all kinds are valuable to both children and elderly people. Children learn 'care' as they attend to their pets' needs, as well as learning facts about animals. Lonely and upset children – of which there are regretfully many in today's stressful society – can gain much comfort from a pet.

A few sensible precautions will, however, need to be taken to ensure that the risk of toxocara infection to young children is reduced to a minimum, as follows.

- Puppies should be wormed regularly with the appropriate medication – available from pharmacists or vets.
- Children should be taught not to allow dogs to lick their faces, and to wash their hands thoroughly after fondling their pets, and certainly always before eating.
- Dog owners should control their dogs at all times, and should not allow them to foul public walk-ways or open spaces.

- Communities should ensure that it is not possible for dogs to foul playing fields, sandpits or other places where children are encouraged to play.

If these precautions are adhered to, toxocara infections could be eliminated without the need to destroy or ban all dogs as pets.

SELF-HELP GROUP

The following group gives information on ways of preventing toxocara infection:

Community Hygiene Concern
32 Crane Avenue
Isleworth
Middlesex TW7 7JL
(Tel. 081 341 7167)

Tuberculosis

INCIDENCE

In developed countries of the world, tuberculosis has reduced rapidly in incidence over the past half century or so. In 1947, 2000 children died from tuberculosis in England and Wales. Forty years later, in the years between 1985 and 1987, just three children died from the disease – a dramatic reduction indeed! This fall is due to better living conditions and less overcrowding as well as better treatment of known cases of tuberculosis. 'Contact tracing', and subsequent treatment if necessary of people having lived or worked in close proximity to a sufferer, has also done much to reduce the incidence of tuberculosis. Nevertheless this infectious disease remains an important problem in Britain, especially amongst immigrant peoples, particularly those from the Indian subcontinent. People living in unhygienic conditions are also at increased risk of contracting this disease.

World-wide the picture is different. It is estimated that every year there are between 3 and 4 million infectious new cases of tuberculosis, with probably an equal number of people having a smear-negative (or non-infectious) tuberculosis. The figure for children suffering from tuberculosis world-wide is around one and a quarter million cases every year. Of these half a million children will die from the disease.

The difference between infectious and non-infectious cases of tuberculosis is important from the point of view of spread of the disease. Infectious cases are those people who cough up the infecting organism, which can thus be passed on to other people – children and adults. These people are known to be 'smear positive', as the offending bacteria can be isolated from their sputum. Non-infectious people can have the disease – in any number of systems of their bodies, including the lungs – but do not cough up the organism. They are therefore known as 'smear negative', as their sputum does not contain the tuberculosis bacillus.

When infection with tuberculosis has occurred, the body becomes sensitive to the protein contained in the bacillus. This sensitivity shows itself in a positive skin reaction when a special preparation of the purified protein derivative (PPD) of the tuberculosis bacteria is injected into the superficial layers of the skin. This is the basis for the Mantoux, Heaf and Tine tests to be described later. Epidemiological data on the number of children showing a positive reaction in 1950, and again in 1990, emphasize further the decline in infection with tuberculosis. In 1950, almost 50% of the 14-year-old children tested were found to be positive, showing that they had met – and overcome – infection with the tuberculosis bacterium. In 1990 less than 1% of children tested in a similar age group were found to be positive.

CAUSATION

Tuberculosis is caused by a bacterium from the mycobacterium group, and was first described by Dr Robert Koch.

As well as tuberculosis being passed on from other human beings, the infection can be transmitted in milk from infected cows. This mode of transmission never occurs in developed countries these days due to the tuberculin testing of all herds of cows to be sure that they are free from this disease.

CHARACTERISTICS

The initial infection with tuberculosis is in the lung. This **primary focus** can subsequently progress in two different ways.

1. On settling in the lungs, the bacteria will multiply here (usually in the upper part of one or other lung). The lymph nodes draining the affected part of the lung will also become involved in the infection. This group of involved tissues is then known as the **primary complex**. This infection can easily pass unnoticed, or occasionally the child will run a low-grade fever and be vaguely off-colour for a week or two. The body's natural defences are mobilized and seal off the infected area of lung. It is at this stage – which is reached within 4–6 weeks – that the skin tests for tuberculosis become positive. The lesion in the lung is usually too small to be visualized on X-ray, although the inflamed lymph nodes around the area can often be seen. This primary infection proceeding along these lines is not infectious to anyone else. Later in life this primary focus can become reactivated. The tuberculosis bacillus can remain dormant for many years. Symptoms can occur when the bacteria are released from their dormant state due to a general lowering of the body's resistance for a variety of reasons – other illness or a general decline in health, for example.)
2. If the child is poorly nourished, ill with another concurrent infection, taking immunosuppressant drugs for some other condition or merely in generally low health, this initial infection with the tuberculosis bacterium can spread, through the blood, to a wide range of other tissues in the body, including other parts of the lung. In the lung extensive destruction

of lung tissue can result and the child will be seriously ill. There will be a **fever**, a **persistent cough** and **night sweats**. Fortunately this picture is rarely encountered in Britain today, but has always to be remembered with this classic triad of symptoms.

The tuberculosis bacillus can invade the **meninges** (the delicate tissue covering the brain and spinal cord), giving rise to tuberculose meningitis. Symptoms of this will be the usual ones of meningitis due to any cause – headache, vomiting and fever. Lumbar pucture is required to obtain a sample of cerebrospinal fluid for laboratory analysis to determine the invading organism causing the symptoms.

Bone can also be affected by the spread of the bacteria. The spine is the most usual site affected, closely followed by knees and/or hips. The affected site will be painful, and X-ray changes will confirm the diagnosis.

Lymph nodes, especially those in the neck, can also be the site to which the tuberculosis bacillus moves. Initially these infected glands will be enlarged but not tender as they are with a throat or ear infection. Later, if untreated, these swollen glands may break down and discharge. (Scars in this region of the neck are not infrequently seen in older people who have had to have these glands operated on.)

Other organs, such as **intestines, kidneys** and **larynx**, can be affected also, but this is rarely seen in children in western countries today.

All these latter aspects of spread from the primary focus are uncommon in developed countries of the world nowadays. But in other parts of the world, where poverty and disease are rife, these problems are not rare.

INVESTIGATIONS

X-ray of the chest, or other parts of the body where suspicious symptoms occur, will show in most cases the typical lesions of tuberculosis.

A **Heaf, Mantoux** or **Tine test** (described later) will also be positive if the infection is due to the tuberculosis bacterium. The extent of the reaction to these tests will point to the range of activity of the infection.

MANAGEMENT

The primary complex is often not treated, as it frequently passes unnoticed. Even if the child is slightly feverish and off-colour for a short while, the true cause of the malaise is rarely discovered. Some authorities suggest that a known primary focus should be treated in order to prevent spread of the disease. (It must be emphasized that this primary focus is not infectious.)

Treatments for other forms of tuberculosis belong to a highly specialized area of medicine. There are a number of **drugs** available for use in tuberculosis infection today. (This is in direct contrast to bygone days when fresh air and good nutrition were the only available treatments.) These drugs will need to be continued for some length of time – up to 1 year to 18 months in order to fully eradicate the disease. The child, of course, must be carefully monitored throughout this time both for success of treatment and for possible adverse side-effects from the drugs used.

Attention to **living conditions** must also be of paramount importance in the successful management of tuberculosis.

Adequate and appropriate **nutrition** of the sick child (and probably the immediate family as well) can also need attention.

Adequate **contact tracing** of other members of the family and other close social contacts must be carefully undertaken.

Schooling can be continued if the child feels well enough to cope with its demands. But arrangements for home tuition may well be necessary during the early stages of treatment depending on the site and severity of the infection.

COMPLICATIONS

These have already been referred to in the generalized spread of tuberculosis.

PREVENTION

BCG vaccination: this vaccine was first produced by the Frenchmen Calmette and Guerin in 1921, the vaccine being named after them. It has been used in England to protect against the spread of tuberculosis since 1948.

In Britain, BCG immunization is recommended for four specific groups:

1. newborn babies who live in households where there is a history of infection with the tuberculosis bacterium;
2. babies born to immigrant families – those people from the Indian subcontinent are particularly at risk and especially so if return visits are made to India where the infection is an ever-present problem;
3. close contacts of people proved to be suffering from active tuberculosis;
4. people whose work leads them into contact with possible sources of tuberculosis, such as health workers and students in teacher training colleges.

In addition to these groups, in Britain BCG vaccine is given to all schoolchildren between the ages of 11 and 13 years. This procedure is regularly under review, as some authorities consider that good contact tracing, followed by either treatment or vaccination, is a preferable way of controlling the spread of infection.

Before the BCG vaccine is given, a Heaf test is performed (the Mantoux test is similar but rarely used today – and the Tine test is used in younger children for its ease of use) 1 week to 10 days previously. This test involves introducing intradermally (usually by means of a special instrument with tiny prongs – the Heaf 'gun') a tiny amount of attenuated tuberculin. This test is done on the inside of the child's arm. The results are read a week later, and graded according to response from 0 to 4 – 0 is equivalent to no response and 4 is equivalent to a reaction over 10 mm in diameter. Grade 2 readings and upwards imply that the child has met the tuberculosis bacillus and has developed immunity. Under these conditions the BCG vaccine will not need to be given. Children with grades 0 and 1 response will need immunization. As mentioned previously, the vast majority of children in Britain today will show this latter reaction.

The BCG vaccination is given intradermally into the upper arm. This will result in a small spot within 2–4 weeks. Sometimes this can ulcerate and discharge, taking up to 3 months to finally heal.

Contraindications to receiving the BCG vaccine are malignancy or an immunological disease, or steroids.

Tuberculosis is an infection against which vigilance must be maintained. In many parts of the world it is still a potent killer, and especially so of late in sufferers with HIV infection. Rapid and adequate tracing of contacts of all cases of known tuberculosis is the first line of defence, with BCG vaccination a close second.

THE FUTURE

Old tuberculosis infection in the lung can be reactivated in later life if, for some reason, the body's defences are reduced. This could be due to adverse physical surroundings, for example, or other illness or infection. It is vital that both the sufferers and their immediate contacts should receive quick and appropriate treatment.

Urinary tract infection

INCIDENCE

Urinary tract infections are more common in childhood than used to be thought a few decades ago. Part of the reason for this is that the signs and symptoms are often so non-specific and intermittent that the condition goes unrecognized.

The prevalence is estimated to be between 1% and 2% in girls, but below 1% in boys. (In infancy this sex difference does not seem to apply, as many boys being affected as are girls.) It is thought that each general practice (of an average of around 10 000 people of all ages) will see at least two or three children every year with a new urinary tract infection. Perhaps this does not seem an enormous number, but nevertheless for the individual child it is important that the diagnosis is made and the condition treated adequately to prevent further problems in later life.

Urinary tract infections can be the first clue given as to the presence of abnormalities in the renal tract. These abnormalities if undiscovered – and hence untreated – can again give rise to problems later in life.

CAUSATION

Urinary tract infections are caused by bacteria. The type of bacteria involved are usually those found normally in the gastrointestinal tract where they do no harm. *E. coli* is one of the commonest types involved. Infection of the renal tract does not usually occur, due to the natural defence mechanisms of the body. For example, any bacteria gaining access to the bladder are regularly washed out by the flow of urine. Also, the child's natural immune defences preclude the infection gaining a hold in the renal tract. (Girls are more at risk from this method of infection than are boys, due to the relative shortness of their urethra.) Breakdown of the natural defence mechanisms can be caused by urine remaining in the bladder for relatively long periods of time. This in turn can be due to a number of factors, as follows.

- There can be **vesico-ureteric reflux**, in which urine is refluxed back into the ureters. Around 40% of children with recurrent urinary tract infections are shown to have this defect on X-ray examination. The phenomenon is thought to have its origins in a congenital defect in the anatomy at the junction of the ureters with the bladder.

- There can be an **obstruction** to the normal outflow of urine from the bladder. Folds, or valves, in the urethra can be a factor causing this type of obstruction, as can stones in older children.
- **Incomplete emptying** of the bladder, due to haste, can also have a bearing on the amount of urine which remains in the bladder for long periods of time. Children are usually impatient to empty their bladders and can be skilled at saying they have 'finished' when, in fact, a great quantity of urine can be remaining in the bladder. (Later, in schooldays, the bladder may be emptied infrequently – perhaps due to a dislike, or fear, of school toilets. This can cause the bladder to overdistend and subsequently to empty incompletely.)

The causative factors in the onset of urinary tract infections are complex and are intricately interwoven. Various tests, interpreted by skilled personnel, are necessary to unravel these factors in each individual child.

CHARACTERISTICS

Urinary tract infections are notoriously difficult to diagnose in children, as signs and symptoms can be vague and non-specific and often apparently unrelated to the urinary tract. The younger the child, the more non-specific will be the symptoms.

Classically, the symptoms associated with a urinary tract infection are:

- **pain** on passing urine – a hot, burning sensation as the urine is voided;
- **pain** in either the lower abdomen, or higher up in the loin region if the infection has reached the kidneys, when it is known as a **pyelonephritis**;
- **frequency** in the passage of urine;
- **enuresis** and/or daytime wetting;
- the passage of **blood** in the urine (haematuria).

This picture is more usually seen in the older child with a urinary infection.

Younger children are more likely to be suffering from a urinary infection when:

- there is a **failure to gain weight** adequately;
- the child is generally **irritable**, especially when this is also associated with a **poor appetite**;
- there is a **low-grade fever**, or spikes of fever with maybe an associated febrile convulsion;

- there is **vomiting** with no previous obvious tummy upset.

Examination of a sample of urine will either confirm, or exclude, a urinary tract infection.

INVESTIGATIONS

Urine testing: it is necessary that a clean sample (i.e. one that is not contaminated with either bacteria from the surrounding skin or faeces) is obtained. To obtain a clean sample the middle of the stream of urine should be taken. This is easier to obtain in boys than in girls without contamination. But with care, and after cleansing of the perineum, a sample can be obtained from a small girl as she sits on the pot or lavatory. Younger children can be fitted with a special bag until sufficient urine is obtained – again, of course, after thorough cleansing of the perineum.

The urine should be examined under the microscope as soon as possible after collection – within an hour if left un-refrigerated. (Refrigeration at 4 °C for 24 hours is satisfactory for later laboratory examination.) Any pus cells, white blood cells and bacteria can be visualized under the microscope if they are present.

A further method – of value in the general practice situation – is to use a special 'dip-slide' (which is a slide coated with a special culture medium). This slide is passed through the stream of urine and subsequently sent to the laboratory.

Blood tests will show a raised white blood cell count and ESR if an infection is present.

If urine testing proves infection to be the cause of the child's symptoms, further investigations (after the treatment of the acute attack) should be done in order to:

- see if the kidneys have been involved in this, or previous, infections;
- detect any abnormalities in the renal tract.

There are a number of specialized tests available. Different authorities usually have preference for one test over another. Also, the investigations pursued in any one individual child will depend on the facilities available locally. These possible investigations include the following.

- **X-ray** examination of the abdomen: this, as a preliminary examination, will exclude any defects in the spine which may be causative factors in the onset of the urinary tract infections. Any calcium stones in the urinary tract will also be shown up by this examination.
- **Ultrasound** investigation: this can detect any obstructive problems as well as being of use in measuring bladder capacity and function.

- A **micturating cystogram** in which a radio-opaque dye is passed up into the bladder. As this is subsequently voided from the bladder, X-ray pictures are taken of the process. This is a particularly useful investigation in the detection of vesico-ureteric reflux. Also, any congenital kidney abnormalities – such as 'horse-shoe' or 'duplex' kidneys – will be detected. Again, the extent of any scarring of the kidneys, from previous infections, can be seen.
- **Isotope scanning** (DMSA scan) is a further investigation that is available at some centres. This specialized investigation is especially valuable in determining the presence and/or extent of kidney damage.
- **Intravenous urography** can also be used, and gives a comprehensive image of the structure and function of the whole urinary tract. This involves an intravenous injection of a radio-opaque substance.

Not all these investigations will, of course, be necessary in any one individual child. Local availability, medical preference and the duration and severity of symptoms will all be taken into account when investigations are planned.

(Regretfully, child sexual abuse must always be remembered in children of all ages with recurrent urinary tract infections, and watch must be kept for other signs and symptoms of this sad situation.)

MANAGEMENT

The acute attack

Babies and children with a severe urinary tract infection will need hospital treatment. Older children and those with a milder attack can be treated at home.

Antibiotics will need to be given as soon as possible. The choice of antibiotic will depend on the type of organism causing the infection. (It is not necessary, or wise, to await laboratory results before starting treatment. A wide-spectrum antibiotic can be used until sensitivities are available. The type of antibiotic can always be changed if it is found that a different one is more satisfactory for the specific infection.) Children who are seriously ill, or who are vomiting frequently, will need to be given antibiotics intravenously. Seven days of antibiotic should clear the infection.

Plenty of **fluids** and an **analgesic** if pain is a problem will help to lower temperature and reduce malaise. (Barley water, available in a variety of commercial flavours, is a useful and palatable drink to give to children. The urine is rendered less acid by these drinks, and provides a less advantageous medium for bacteria.)

'Bubble bath' additives should be avoided in the baths of children susceptible to urinary tract infections. The surface tension-lowering action of these additives aids the entry of bacteria into the bladder.

Future management will depend on the results of the investigations undertaken. For example, if any obstruction to the flow of urine, such as stones, is found, this will need to be dealt with. Further infections must be avoided as far as possible to avoid long-term effects. This can be done in the following ways.

- Giving a long-term dose of antibiotic: the length of time that these drugs should be given is variable, but a minimum of 2 years is advised by most authorities.
- Being sure that the child empties the bladder fully: this can be helped by drinking plenty of water, allowing adequate time for visits to the lavatory and by avoiding constipation. (Overloading of the large bowel can exert pressure on the lower urinary tract, and effectively prevent adequate bladder emptying.)

Follow-up appointments to assess progress, with further investigative procedures when necessary, are vital to be sure that a low-grade infection does not continue as well as to encourage child and parents to persist with treatment. Long-term medication can be trying for everyone concerned.

COMPLICATIONS

Recurrent urinary tract infections, with the continuing risk of further renal damage, are an ever-present worry.

Long-term effects, which will become evident in later life, are **renal failure** if damage has been severe in childhood, and a **high blood pressure** which can also be a late result of kidney problems in childhood. Kidney function is intimately tied up with hypertension, but by early adequate treatment of urinary tract infections in childhood at least one possible cause of this problem can be eliminated.

Urinary tract infections in childhood are an excellent example of how adult disease often has its basis during the early growing years.

Warts

Alternative name

Verrucae.

INCIDENCE

Warts are common skin lesions and especially so during childhood. In fact, almost all children will have warts somewhere on their bodies before adulthood is reached.

Verrucae – or plantar warts – found on children's feet reach almost epidemic proportions at times. This type of wart is rarely seen after the age of 16 years.

HISTORY

Warts have been referred to in history from time immemorial. Probably one of the best known characters in British history with facial warts is Oliver Cromwell, who had a splendid crop.

It is only in recent years that a greater interest has been shown in these benign tumours of the skin. The causative factor – a particular type of virus – is known and is seen to multiply rapidly in the nuclei of cells. It is recognized that, under certain circumstances, infection with one of the viruses causing warts can lead to malignant change. Further study of warts may help to unravel aspects of malignancies in the body.

CAUSATION

Warts are caused by one of the papilloma viruses – of which there are many – of the papova group. It is thought that the incubation period (the period between infection and the appearance of the wart) is long.

CHARACTERISTICS

Four different types of wart are described and, although these can over-lap, it is possible that a different subgroup of virus is involved in each type.

The **common wart** or **verruca vulgaris** is most usually seen over bony surfaces such as knees and elbows. It is possible that small, regular episodes of minor injury to these parts of the body allow the virus to gain a hold. These warts are raised and under a magnifying lens can be seen to have an irregular, bumpy surface.

Plane warts are, as their name implies, flat and are usually found on exposed parts of the body, particularly the face. They are also seen to occur along the margins of scratches and cuts – frequently in large numbers.

Plantar warts – usually referred to merely as 'verrucae' – are found on the soles of the feet. Over recent years much publicity has been given to this type of wart in relation to the high number of children acquiring verrucae from swimming baths and also following barefoot exercise and dancing. They can become large and exceedingly painful due to the trauma of continually walking on them.

Warts around the **anus** and **genital regions** of the body tend to have a frilly, fronded appearance. Sexual abuse must always be borne in mind when a child is found to have warts on this part of the body.

MANAGEMENT

This can be fraught with difficulties due to a number of factors.

- The position of the warts: for example, numerous plane warts on the face can be very difficult to treat. Plantar warts, too, can be numerous and cover a large, much-used part of the foot. Numerous warts on fingers can also cause problems by getting in the way of fine, delicate activities.
- The fact that warts frequently occur in groups makes treatment difficult.
- Warts quickly appear out of the blue, and at times disappear with equal rapidity. (Many are the old wives' tales of this phenomenon – one of the best known being to rub the wart with raw steak and then bury the steak in the garden. As the meat degenerates, so, too, will the wart disappear!)

Specific treatments include the following.

- **Paints**, which basically remove hard skin, can be applied to the wart on a regular daily basis. It is preferable that the painted area is covered by a plaster dressing to avoid the paint being rubbed off. This treatment will need to be continued for some time, and frequently fails due to its long-term nature.

- **Podophyllin** can be used for single or a few warts. Again this should be applied daily and covered with a dressing. This substance must be used with caution, however, as it is extremely irritant when applied to normal skin. Between applications, the surface of the wart can be gently rubbed away.

Both the above preparations can be bought over the counter in main pharmacists.

Carbon dioxide 'snow' or **liquid nitrogen** can also be used for isolated warts. Again it is important that the wart should be treated accurately, as surrounding normal skin can be easily damaged.

Soaking the feet daily in a **solution of formaldehyde** used to be a favourite treatment for verrucae. Following each 'soak', the surface of the wart was gently pared away. Once again this is slow, long-term treatment, and is rarely used today.

Warts can be **cauterized**. A little local anaesthetic is injected around the wart and the warty tissue burnt away. Care must be taken not to damage the surrounding skin. It is unwise to use this method for warts arising over joints or on the palms of the hands or soles of the feet. The resultant scars can be painful in these specific locations.

A simple, but often effective, method for the solitary wart is merely to cover it with an **airtight plaster**. This effectively cuts off the oxygen supply to the wart. After 2 or 3 weeks of this treatment – changing the plaster at bath-times, or as and when it becomes dirty or loose – the wart will become soft and friable. It can then be gently scrubbed off with pumice or an ordinary nail-brush.

PREVENTION

Preventative methods are only possible with plantar warts – the ubiquitous verrucae that are passed so readily from child to child in the warm, moist atmosphere of swimming baths. A few authorities still inspect children's feet before swimming and follow this by exclusion from the baths of those children found to have a verruca. This is difficult to implement fully, and perhaps not entirely reasonable to enforce. No child ever died from a verruca, but many children have lost their lives through being unable to swim.

Verruca socks have had their vogue in the past and are still available. Children don these foot coverings before entering the changing room (where most of the infections are passed on) of swimming baths.

Warts are a nuisance rather than being dangerous. But there are occasions when treatment for these irritating lesions becomes necessary. Painful verrucae on feet, disfiguring marks on the face or warts on fingers getting in the way of daily activities are all examples of reasons for active treatment. But even with conscientious treatment, warts can be particularly persistent. Their only saving grace is that they will eventually disappear spontaneously within a year or two if left alone!

Whooping cough

Alternative names

Pertussis.
The 'cough of a hundred days'.

INCIDENCE

The incidence of whooping cough in England and Wales has shown a marked variation over the past 25 years. This is closely related to the uptake of whooping cough vaccine; the incidence dramatically increased when immunization rates were low, and fell again as immunization against this vicious disease became more acceptable.

Pertussis (whooping cough) is known world-wide, and estimated figures in 1986 were 60 million cases in a year. Half a million deaths annually were also reported at this time. Without immunization, it is thought that by the age of 5 years 80% of children are infected. Whooping cough is unusual amongst the childhood infections in being more common in girls, and also of greater severity.

Epidemics of this infection occur once every 3–4 years. This has been noted both in the UK and in other countries where reports of infectious disease are relatively reliable. (It is thought that whooping cough is under-reported in most countries where standardized reporting systems are in place. So the true incidence of this disease is probably very high indeed.) This 3–4 year pattern was noticed again in Britain when the immunization figures fell to a low level in the 1970s. During the 10 years or so that it took for the immunization levels to rise again, two epidemics were noted – in 1978–1979 and 1982–1983. At both these times over 400 000 cases were notified.

CAUSATION

Whooping cough is caused by a bacterium. This bacterium is spread by droplet infection from a child already suffering from the disease.

The mode of action of the whooping cough bacterium (*Bordetella pertussis*) is unusual. The bacterium itself attacks, first of all, the respiratory passages, producing the initial symptoms of the disease, which are rather similar to those of a common cold. The bacterium then produces a toxin which attacks various cells throughout the body. So whilst the initial bacterial attack is susceptible to – and can be treated with – antibiotics, these drugs will have no effect on the later toxin.

The incubation period of whooping cough is 7–14 days, 10 days being the average time before the next family member starts to show symptoms.

CHARACTERISTICS

Whooping cough is a long illness, with three distinct phases, as follows.

1. During the **catarrhal** stage, symptoms closely akin to those of a common cold occur – a **runny nose**, a **cough** and a mild **fever**. This stage can be so comparatively mild that the child may still be at school or playing with peers. As the child is infectious at this time, the disease can be quickly spread.

2. The **paroxysmal** stage follows after about 10 days. This is when the cough occurs in severe spasms with the child having great difficulty in getting adequate breath between the paroxysms. The face will become puce and even blue with the effort to get air into the lungs, and the paroxysm will end in a 'whoop' as the air is finally drawn in a rush into the lungs. Once the 'whoop' of whooping cough has been heard it can never be forgotten. **Vomiting** frequently occurs at the end of the paroxysm of coughing, particularly if the child has just eaten. These paroxysmal attacks are extremely distressing to both parent and child. With closely repeated paroxysms the whole family – and especially the sufferer – can become completely exhausted. This phase can last up to a fortnight. The lack of oxygen experienced by the child during these paroxysms of coughing can be the cause of one of the most serious of the complications seen due to whooping cough. The severity of these paroxysms of coughing can result in **haemorrhages** into various parts of the body – into the conjunctiva of the eyes, from the nose and even small bleeding areas into the skin.

3. During the **convalescent** stage, the cough gradually decreases in both frequency and severity, but can still be in evidence up to 3 months later – hence 'the hundred day cough'.

If the disease occurs in a young baby, the characteristic 'whoop' is often absent. At this age the baby will not have the strength to take the large gasp which is the cause of the typical 'whoop'.

INVESTIGATIONS

The diagnosis of whooping cough is essentially a clinical one, and a very obvious one once the 'whoop' is heard. If there is a current epidemic of whooping cough and a child has a persistent, worsening cough lasting for longer than 2 weeks, whooping cough can be strongly suspected.

Blood tests will show a non-specific increase in certain of the white blood cells.

Laboratory tests on the secretions obtained from the back of the nose and throat can confirm the diagnosis. This, however, is rarely done, partly due to the unpleasantness of the procedure for the child in obtaining a sample of these secretions, and partly due to the unreliability of some of these tests.

MANAGEMENT

A specific **antibiotic**, erythromycin, is given to destroy the bacteria (but has no action against the toxin produced). This treatment will also render the child non-infectious after around 5 days, although the erythromycin should be continued for 2 weeks to be sure of eradicating all the bacteria.

During the unpleasant paroxysmal phase, the child can be helped in a number of ways, as follows.

- Efforts can be made to **avoid** provoking the paroxysms of coughing. For example, sudden changes of temperature can initiate an attack. So nursing in a warm, evenly controlled environment can be helpful. Similarly, bland food which does not irritate the back of the child's throat should be offered.
- **Meals** should be small and frequent. If a fit of coughing results in vomiting with the loss of most of the previous meal, food can be offered again once the attack is over. (Unlike after the vomiting due to a tummy upset, the child will often be willing to eat again immediately after an attack of coughing.) It is important to do all that is possible to maintain the child's **nutrition** during the illness. **Fluids** should also be available in abundance to be sure that dehydration does not complicate the illness.
- The **sticky mucus** produced as part of this disease must be removed from the child's respiratory passages as much as possible. This is especially important in babies and young children who find it difficult, or impossible, to cough up this mucus. (This aspect is one of the reasons why whooping cough is such a dangerous illness in the young child.)
- Children with whooping cough can become very distressed and frightened during the paroxysms of coughing (as can the adults watching their child fighting for breath) and will need much **reassurance**.

Most older children can be **nursed at home** through an attack of whooping cough. Young babies, or those children in difficult or unsuitable home circumstances, will need to be admitted to hospital during the worst of the illness. Hospital admission for a short time may also be necessary to relieve parents who are nursing several children through this long, drawn-out illness.

School can be recommenced as soon as the child feels well enough – as long as at least 5 days' treatment with erythromycin have been given. It is unlikely, however, that the child will feel well enough to return to school for at least 2 or 3 weeks with even a mild attack of whooping cough. Teachers should be fully informed about the **course** of the illness – mainly because the cough, which can last for up to 3 months, can give rise to concern. Teaching staff should be reassured that the child is not infectious during this convalescent stage as long as erythromycin has been given.

COMPLICATIONS

As well as it being a highly unpleasant, and potentially fatal, illness, complications are common with an attack of whooping cough.

Lungs

Bronchopneumonia not infrequently occurs along with an attack of whooping cough. Resistance is lowered by the effects of the whooping cough bacteria and the toxin produced, so that secondary infection is common. If this occurs the child's general condition will deteriorate and there will be a rise in temperature. Treatment will be with a further antibiotic.

Children who suffer from **asthma** will have added problems if they contract whooping cough. Indeed, this infection may bring a hitherto undiagnosed asthma to light. Once recovery from the whooping cough has occurred, appropriate treatment for the asthma must be given. (See 'Asthma'.) Some authorities consider that an attack of asthma in childhood contributes to long-term damage to the lungs, **bronchiecstasis** being a common sequel. Appropriate antibiotic treatment during the acute attack will do much to reduce this possibility.

Ears

Secondary bacterial infection giving rise to **otitis media** is frequently found to occur during the acute stages of whooping cough. Earache and a rise in temperature will give warning of this complication.

Haemorrhages

Due to excessive strain put on blood vessels during the paroxysms of coughing, haemorrhages into various parts of the body can readily occur. Conjunctival haemorrhages, petechiae (bleeding from small blood vessels under the skin) and nose bleeds have already been mentioned. Coughing up of blood from the respiratory passages can also occur and add to parental anxieties.

These haemorrhages will all resolve spontaneously, although nose bleeding can sometimes be a problem to control. Haemoptysis (coughing up of blood) should always be reported to the doctor.

Herniae

Again due to the severity of the paroxysmal attacks of coughing, the pressure inside the abdominal cavity is raised. If there is already a hernia present – in boys most usually in the groin area – or there is an incipient weakness in the muscles in this part of the body, an attack of whooping cough can bring this to light.

Nervous system

It is the complications in the nervous system due to the whooping cough bacterium that are the most serious. These complications can result in long-term handicap. It is thought that there are two ways in which these complications can occur. These are:

1. as a result of the temporary oxygen lack to the tissues, including nervous tissue, from the paroxysms of coughing – anyone who has seen the cyanosis (blueness) of a child's face during a paroxysm will readily understand how tissues are starved of oxygen during those few minutes;
2. as a direct result of the action of the toxin produced by the whooping cough bacteria on nervous tissue.

These neurological complications can manifest themselves as **convulsions** or **loss of consciousness**. If severe, the outcome can be permanent brain damage, resulting in a range of possible effects, including **paralysis, intellectual handicap** and **death**.

Regretfully, there is no treatment that can prevent such tragedies occurring, apart from, of course, earlier prevention by immunization with whooping cough vaccine.

PREVENTION

Whooping cough can be prevented by immunization with whooping cough vaccine. This vaccine is offered, in Britain, as part of the routine baby-hood immunization schedule, and is given together with vaccines against diphtheria and tetanus as the 'triple' vaccine at 2, 3 and 4 months of age. If the whooping cough part of this triple vaccine has been missed out for any reason, it can be given as three doses of single whooping cough vaccine at monthly intervals.

Contraindications to receiving this vaccine are few.

- If the child has a feverish illness when any immunization procedures are due, they should be postponed until recovery has taken place, and this, of course, applies to the whooping cough vaccine as much as any other.
- If there has been a **severe** generalized reaction to a previous dose of the whooping cough vaccine, this part of the triple vaccine should be omitted in future. A severe reaction means a high fever (over 39.5°C) within 48 hours of the injection, convulsions, anaphylactic shock or prolonged, inconsolable screaming by the baby within 72 hours of the injection being given. These are all pretty dramatic occurrences which should not be confused with mild reactions such as a slight fever or irritability for a few hours. These latter mild reactions can occur following immunization with the whooping cough vaccine. But when compared with the possible effects of a naturally acquired attack of whooping cough, the benefits of immunization can be seen.
- If there has been a **severe** local reaction to a previous immunization at the site of the actual injection – this means a large area of redness and swelling, covering the front and side of the baby's thigh or much of the circumference of the arm, depending on where the injection has been given – vaccine should not be given.

Asthma or eczema are not contraindications to receiving the whooping cough vaccine, and no child should be denied the protection of this vaccine due to suffering from these conditions. If the baby has had any convulsions earlier in life, or there is a strong history of epilepsy in the immediate family, individual advice regarding this must be taken from a doctor specializing in immunization problems.

THE FUTURE

For the individual, late effects of an attack of whooping cough will depend on any complications that may have occurred. For most children an attack of whooping cough will be a dim, distant, albeit unpleasant, memory. But for some unfortunate children, this infection will colour the whole of the rest of their lives.

Appendix A
The progress of infectious diseases (uncomplicated)

INTRODUCTION

It must be emphasized that as no two people are the same, and the same disease affects people in different ways, the following information should only be treated as a guide.

CHICKENPOX

Days	Stage	Comments
	Incubation	14–17 days
1–5	Rash crops	Crops of 'blistery' spots arise every 2–3 days
1–6	Fever	Usually peaks on third day – can be up to 39°C
6–9	Rash scabs	Spots crust over

NB. All stages of the rash can be seen at the same time.

MEASLES

Days	Stage	Comments
	Incubation	10–14 days
1–7	Conjunctivitis	Sore reddened eyes associated with photophobia
1–7	Fever	Up to 40°C – usually peaks on fourth day
1–7	Coryza	
1–11	Cough	Harsh dry cough
2–6	Koplik's spots	To be found on inside of cheeks opposite the back molars – similar to grains of salt
4–9	Rash – discrete	Face, upper torso and arms – becoming a confluent dense rash all over the body after about 1–3 days

RUBELLA

Days	Stage	Comments
	Incubation	14–21 days
1–8	Malaise	
1–12	Lymph nodes	Tender enlarged glands at back of neck
4–7	Conjunctivitis	Mild only, with no photophobia
4–7	Coryza	
4–7	Rash	Fine, pink discrete spots
5–8	Fever	Mild only, but may be up to 38°C on fifth day

SCARLET FEVER

Days	Stage	Comments
	Incubation	2–4 days
1–5	Sore throat	**Severe** sore throat
2–7	Fever	Can be up to 40°C on third day
2–7	Rash	Bright scarlet in colour

Appendix B
Glossary

Abdominal cavity	That part of the torso below the diaphragm, containing many important organs.
Aetiology	The cause of, or factors involved in, the onset of a disease.
Alveoli	Lung tissue involved in gaseous exchange.
Anal fissure	Crack in skin around anus.
Analgesics	Pain-relieving drugs.
Androgens	Male sex hormones.
Anorexia	Loss of appetite.
Antibiotics	Drugs active against bacterial infections.
Anus	Ring of muscular tissue at lower end of large bowel.
Auroscope	Instrument used for examining ears.
Capillaries	The smallest blood vessels in the body.
Cataract	Clouding of the lens of the eye.
Cellulitis	Widespread inflammation of connective tissue.
Cerebrospinal fluid	Fluid surrounding the brain and spinal cord.
Chorea	Involuntary, non-stereotyped muscular movements.
Chromosomes	Units in every cell on which genes are situated.
Chronic	Long-standing.
Comedomes	Plugs of hard skin found in acne.
Congenital	Conditions present at or from birth, with developmental origin implied.
Conjunctiva	Delicate tissue covering the eye.
Conjunctivitis	Inflammation of the conjunctiva.
Connective tissue	Tissues surrounding all the organs of the body.
Constitutional upset	Generalized illness, usually with fever and malaise.
CT scan	Computer-aided tomography.
Desquamation	Peeling of the superficial layers of the skin.
Developmental checks	Standardized tests used to check childhood development.

Diaphragm	Strong sheet of muscle dividing the abdominal cavity from the chest cavity.
Dietician	Personnel trained in nutrition.
Droplet infection	Spread of infection from minute drops of secretions in a person's breath.
EEG	Electroencephalogram.
Elimination diets	Diets used to exclude possible cause of an allergy.
Emollient creams	Greasy ointments or creams used in treatment of skin diseases.
Encephalitis	Inflammation of the brain.
Epicanthic folds	Folds of skin over inner surface of some children's eyes.
Epistaxis	Nose bleeding.
ESR	Erythrocyte sedimentation rate – laboratory test used as an indicator of an infective process.
Erythromycin	A particular type of antibiotic.
Eustachian tube	Tiny tube linking the middle ear with the back of the throat.
Febrile convulsions	Convulsions (fits or seizures) seen in children under the age of 5 years due to a sudden rise in temperature.
Glaucoma	Condition in which pressure inside the eye is raised.
Glycosuria	Sugar in the urine.
Haematuria	Blood in the urine.
Haemoglobin	Substance in red blood cells carrying oxygen.
Haemophilia	Condition associated with clotting of blood.
Haemoptysis	Coughing up of blood.
Hernia	Weakness in muscular wall – usually of abdomen.
Hirschsprung's disease	Condition in which there are narrowed segments of bowel.
Hormones	Internal secretions produced by endocrine or ductless glands that exercise a specific physiological effect on a target organ, to which they are carried by the blood.
Hypoglycaemia	Low blood sugar.
Hypothermia	Low body temperature.
Immunization	Procedures eliciting a response in the body which protects against specific infections met at a later date.
Immunosuppressed	A procedure whereby the immune system is suppressed by drugs in the treatment of certain diseases.

Incubation period	That period of time between exposure to an infection and the onset of symptoms.
Inhaler	Specialized equipment used to introduce medication into the lungs.
Jaundice	Yellow coloration of the skin due to malfunction of the liver.
Ketones	Substances which can arise from the breakdown of body tissue.
Koplik spots	Spots seen on inside of cheeks in the early stages of measles.
Labyrinthitis	Inflammation of structures inside the ears due to infection, causing giddiness.
Lumbar puncture	Procedure whereby cerebrospinal fluid is withdrawn for diagnostic purposes.
Lymph nodes	Congregation of lymph tissue in many different parts of the body.
Malaise	General feeling of illness.
Mastoid process	Bony projection of skull behind and below the ears.
Menarche	Time of onset of menstruation in girls at puberty.
Meninges	Thin, delicate covering of brain and spinal cord.
Meningitis	Inflammation of meninges.
Myringotomy	Procedure whereby an opening is made in the eardrum to withdraw fluid from the middle ear.
Nebulizer	Equipment for introducing medication into lungs by way of a face mask.
Oestrogens	Female sex hormones.
Orchitis	Inflammation of the testes.
Ossicles	Tiny bones in the middle ear – three in number.
Osteoporosis	Reduction in density of bones.
Pancreatitis	Inflammation of the pancreas.
Parasite	An organism living off another organism.
Parotid glands	Salivary glands situated in front of, and below, the ears.
Parotitis	Inflammation of the parotid salivary glands.
Petechiae	Small bleeding points under the skin.
Photophobia	Dislike of light.
Pica	Eating of dirt or other unsuitable substances, e.g. coal, chalk.
Psychiatrist	A doctor specializing in mental illness.
Refractive error	Errors in the bending of light onto the retina.
Renal tract	Organs of excretion, consisting of kidneys, ureters, bladder and urethra.

Retina	The structure at the back of the eye intimately concerned with vision.
Rheumatoid factor	Factor found in the blood of sufferers from some kinds of rheumatism or arthritis.
Rickets	Disease of bone due to lack of calcium and/or vitamin D.
Scoliosis	Sideways twist to the spine.
Sebaceous glands	Glands found all over the body producing sebum, which gives the skin its oily nature.
Septicaemia	Blood poisoning.
Signing	Language using hand movements for deaf people.
Soft palate	Back of the roof of the mouth.
Syndrome	A combination of signs and symptoms which, when put together, form a recognizable pattern.
Tonsils	Aggregations of lymphoid tissue on either side of the throat.
Toxin	Substance produced by certain bacteria.
Trachea	Windpipe.
Ureters	Tubes connecting kidneys to bladder.
Urethra	Passage from bladder to exterior.
Vasculitis	Inflammation of the small blood vessels.

Further reading

Carson, P. (1987) *Coping Successfully with your Child's Asthma*, Sheldon Press, London.

David, T.J. (ed.) (1992) *Recent Advances in Paediatrics*, Churchill Livingstone, Edinburgh.

Department of Health, Welsh Ofice (1992) *Immunisation against Infectious Disease*, HMSO Publications, London.

Elliott, J. (1987) *If Your Child is Diabetic*, Sheldon Press, London.

Forfar, J.O. (ed.) (1988) *Child Health in a Changing Society*, Oxford University Press, Oxford.

Hall, D.M.B. (1989) *Health for All Children*, Oxford Medical Publishers, Oxford.

Knight, A. (1981) *Asthma and Hay-fever*, Positive Health Guides, London.

Lewis, S. and National Eczema Society (1994) *The Eczema Handbook*, Vermilion, London.

Nicoll, A. (ed.) (1989) *Manual on Infections and Immunisations in Children*, Oxford Medical Publications, Oxford.

Palmar, R.L. (1989) *Anorexia Nervosa*, Penguin Books, London.

Polney, L. (1989) *Manual of Community Paediatrics*, Churchill Livingsone, Edinburgh.

Reisner, H. (1987) *Children with Epilepsy*, Woodbine House, Rockville, USA.

Rossiter, J. and Seddon, R. (1992) *Diabetic Kid's Cookbook*, Positive Health Guides, London.

Taitz, L.S. and Wardley, B. (1989) *Handbook of Child Nutrition*, Oxford Medical Publishers, Oxford.

van Riel, P. (1987) *Acne*, Sheldon Press, London.

Index